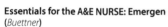 **OTHER *ESSENTIALS* BO**

CW00796730

Essentials for the NEW NURSE PRACTITI
Nutshell (*Aktan*)

Essentials for the A&E NURSE: Emergen
(*Buettner*)

Essentials About GI AND LIVER DISEASES FOR NURSES: What APRNs Need to Know in a Nutshell (*Chaney*)

Essentials on COMBATTING NURSE BULLYING, INCIVILITY, AND WORKPLACE VIOLENCE: What Nurses Need to Know in a Nutshell (*Ciocco*)

Essentials for the THEATRE NURSE: An Orientation and Care Guide in a Nutshell (*Criscitelli*)

Essentials for the NEONATAL NURSE: A Nursing Orientation and Care Guide in a Nutshell (*Davidson*)

Essentials for the LONG-TERM CARE NURSE: What Nursing Home and Assisted Living Nurses Need to Know in a Nutshell (*Eliopoulos*)

Essentials for the CLINICAL NURSE MANAGER: Managing a Changing Workplace in a Nutshell (*Fry*)

Essentials for EVIDENCE-BASED PRACTICE: Implementing EBP in a Nutshell (*Godshall*)

Essentials for Nurses About HOME INFUSION THERAPY: The Expert's Best Practice Guide in a Nutshell (*Gorski*)

Essentials for MIDWIVES: Labour & Delivery Orientation in a Nutshell (*Groll*)

Essentials for the RADIOLOGY NURSE: An Orientation and Nursing Care Guide in a Nutshell (*Grossman*)

Essentials for the CARDIAC SURGERY NURSE: Caring for Cardiac Surgery Patients in a Nutshell (*Hodge*)

Essentials for DEMENTIA CARE: What Nurses Need to Know in a Nutshell (*Miller*)

Essentials for STROKE CARE NURSING: An Expert Guide in a Nutshell (*Morrison*)

Essentials for the PAEDIATRIC NURSE: An Orientation Guide in a Nutshell (*Rupert, Young*)

Essentials for the TRIAGE NURSE: An Orientation and Care Guide in a Nutshell (*Visser, Montejano, Grossman*)

Essentials for the HOSPICE NURSE: A Concise Guide to End-of-Life Care (*Wright*)

Essentials About PTSD: A Guide for Nurses and Other Health Care Professionals (*Adams*)

Essentials for the CLINICAL NURSING INSTRUCTOR: Clinical Teaching in a Nutshell (*Kan, Stabler-Haas*)

ESSENTIALS for
THE CATH LAB NURSE

Margarita Berrocal

Brenda Kirkpatrick McCulloch, RN, MSN, RCIS, has been a cardiovascular clinical nurse specialist, supporting the cardiovascular service line at Sutter Medical Center in Sacramento, California, for the past 15 years. Prior to this, she worked in the cath labs at Mercy General Hospital and the University of California-Davis Medical Center, both located in Sacramento. She received her master's degree in nursing from the University of San Francisco, her bachelor's degree in healthcare administration from St. Mary's College in Moraga, California, and her nursing diploma from the Burge School of Nursing in Springfield, Missouri.

Ms. McCulloch has published multiple articles related to cardiovascular nursing in *AORN, Critical Care Nurse, AACN Advanced Critical Care, Critical Care Nursing Clinics*, and *Cath Lab Digest*. She contributed three chapters to the third edition of *Invasive Cardiology: A Manual for Cath Lab Personnel* and was the cardiovascular nursing section editor for the second edition of *Medical-Surgical Nursing*, by Kathleen Osborn, Cheryl Wraa, Annita Watson, and Renee Holleran.

Ms. McCulloch is a member of the American Association of Critical Care Nurses and is a lifetime member of the Sacramento Area Chapter of AACN, having served as chapter president, seminar coordinator, and then newsletter editor for 20 years. She is also a member of the National Association of Clinical Nurse Specialists and was recognized as Clinical Nurse Specialist of the Year in 2013.

ESSENTIALS for
THE CATH LAB NURSE

Brenda Kirkpatrick McCulloch, RN, MSN, RCIS

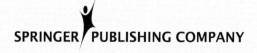

SPRINGER PUBLISHING COMPANY

Springer Publishing Company, LLC
11 West 42nd Street
New York, NY 10036
www.springerpub.com

Acquisitions Editor: Elizabeth Nieginski
Compositor: Amnet Systems

ISBN: 978-0-8261-6131-4

Contact us to receive discount rates on bulk purchases.
We can also customize our books to meet your needs.
For more information, please contact sales@springerpub.com

The ESSENTIALS series was published in the United States by Springer Publishing Company, LLC, as the FAST FACTS series.

Contents

Preface

The cardiac catheterization laboratory (cath lab) is an increasingly complex environment with increasingly challenging procedures. When I was a new graduate nurse, a long time ago, working nights in the cardiac intensive care unit (CICU), patients admitted with an acute ST-segment elevation myocardial infarction (STEMI) did not go to the cath lab; they were hospitalized for at least two weeks. We didn't let patients have cold drinks, we cut up their food for them, and they couldn't have coffee. If they developed heart failure, all we really had for treatment was furosemide and digoxin; beta-blockers were still considered a no-no for heart failure. They had an 80% mortality rate if they developed cardiogenic shock. Today, STEMI patients are taken directly to the cath lab for immediate revascularization with percutaneous coronary intervention within 90 minutes of arrival to the hospital and are discharged within two to three days.

I fell in love with the cath lab in the early 1980s when I transferred there. I had worked almost seven years in critical care and wanted an opportunity to learn new skills. When I first started, there were limited educational resources written for the nurse or technologist working in the cath lab. It was literally a "watch one, do one, teach one" experience. I remember hours of reading from the second edition of Dr. William Grossman's classic textbook *Cardiac Catheterization and Angiography*, published in 1980 (now in its eighth edition), trying to absorb what I could. Since that time, I've become passionate about helping others become more knowledgeable about working in the cath lab.

I was a beginner in the cath lab when coronary balloon angioplasty was introduced in the United States. An angioplasty could take eight hours, while a full cardiac surgery crew sat nearby, waiting to see if they needed to finish what we started. Today, we can complete four trans-catheter aortic valve replacement procedures in an eight-hour day.

I have worked in and around cath labs ever since, as a staff nurse, department coordinator, manager, service line director, and now as a clinical nurse specialist, which I often refer to as the best job in the world. In my 40-year career as a registered nurse, I've seen tremendous growth in cardiology and the birth of a new subspecialty—interventional cardiology. It's been quite a ride!

This book is written from a nursing framework because that is what I know best. I've had the great opportunity to work with great cath lab nurses and technologists and learn from all of them. I fully understand and deeply appreciate that it takes an interdisciplinary team to work most effectively in the cath lab. This interdisciplinary team also includes cardiologists, cardiothoracic surgeons, anesthesiologists, radiology technologists, cardiovascular technologists, echocardiography technologists, and support staff. In the cath lab, all roles are essential and all contribute to patient care and successful procedural outcomes. The whole is always greater than the sum of its parts, as Aristotle observed centuries ago.

Essentials for the Cath Lab Nurse is designed for the nurse new to the cath lab who has some prior experience with cardiovascular patients and can interpret rhythm strips and understand the basics of hemodynamics and cardiovascular medications. Various topics and procedures are included. It is my hope that this book will help the new nurse while building knowledge and confidence. The cath is a dynamic environment and it presents a great opportunity to learn new skills.

- Chapters are designed to progressively walk you through how procedures are completed.
- Each chapter begins with key learning objectives.
- Detailed information about each phase of the procedure is provided.
- A feature called "Essential Facts" provides a quick summary of key points to know.
- When appropriate, a quick anatomy review is provided.

In summary, this handbook is an important orientation resource. You may choose to read it from beginning to end or keep it hand at work as a quick resource before starting a case. While this book cannot contain all the information you need to work successfully in the cath lab setting, my hope is that it will provide a solid base on which you build as you gain experience.

Brenda Kirkpatrick McCulloch

Acknowledgments

I want to thank and acknowledge the many cardiologists, cardio-thoracic surgeons, nurses, technologists, and support staff I've had the privilege to work with throughout my long career in cardio-vascular nursing. They taught me so much about cardiology and about the spirit of great teamwork. I am deeply appreciative of the late Dr. Charles Inlow, the first cardiologist I worked with as a new graduate in Springdale, Arkansas. His knowledge, wisdom, humor, and down-home approach to patient care spurred my fascination with cardiology. He taught me so much about the heart—with great heart. My most sincere appreciation to Dr. Reginald Low of Sacramento, who, so many years ago, walked and talked me through my first scrubbing experience on my fourth day in the cath lab at Mercy General Hospital. Thirty-plus years later, I continue to learn from him and the many cardiologists he has mentored during their fellowships.

Much gratitude to my many amazing colleagues from the cardiovascular service lines of Sutter Medical Center, Mercy General Hospital, and UC Davis Medical Center in Sacramento for your ongoing support. Thanks to the many nurses I have precepted in the cath lab setting. Thanks to the hundreds of nurses and technologists I have interacted with the past 25 years in consulting roles and while teaching in Cath Lab and Beyond, an ongoing educational opportunity offered by the Continuing Education Consortium of Sacramento. Your enthusiasm and inquisitive minds always motivate me to learn and share more. A big thank-you also to Tanya Hodge, my friend and colleague, who wrote *Essentials for the Cardiac Surgery Nurse* and gave me the contact information I needed to get started with this process.

Deep gratitude for my family who have tolerated and supported my work, school, and on-call schedules for decades: my husband, Craig—"just three pages a day"—and our daughter, Megan, an attorney who knows more about cath labs than she wishes she did. I could not have successfully completed this book without your love, support, and thoughtful editing recommendations.

1

The Cath Lab Environment

Cardiac catheterization laboratories, commonly referred to as cath labs, have been in existence for over 50 years and are found in hospitals and in freestanding outpatient settings. Originally, few procedures other than diagnostic testing were performed. In today's cath lab, the list of possible procedures can be extensive and include coronary stenting, peripheral intervention, and catheter-based structural heart repair.

In this chapter, you will learn:

1. Procedures commonly performed in the cath lab
2. Equipment that can be found in the cath lab environment
3. Traditional roles of the cath lab team and the need for effective teamwork
4. Working within a surgical environment

PROCEDURES DONE IN THE CATH LAB

Procedures done in the cath lab setting include:

- Right and left heart catheterization
- Angiography of the coronary arteries, left ventricle, and aorta
- Coronary and peripheral intervention, including balloon angioplasty and stenting

- Transcatheter repairs for structural heart disease, including defect closures and valve intervention
- Pacemaker and device placement

CATH LAB ENVIRONMENT

Cath labs vary significantly among hospitals. In small hospitals, there may be just one procedure room while large medical centers will have multiple procedure rooms. The standard cath lab procedural space needs to be large enough to accommodate the following:

- X-ray system
- Physiologic monitoring system
- Automated power injector
- Multiple display monitors
- Defibrillator
- Carts and cabinets for routine supplies and equipment
- Workstations for the team members

A newer type of cath lab procedure room is the "hybrid" room that combines the high-quality imaging capabilities and hemodynamic monitoring components of the cath lab with an operating room. Hybrid rooms are used for complex procedures that may require both interventional and surgical techniques such as:

- Transcatheter valve replacement
- Endovascular aortic procedures
- Pacemaker lead extractions
- Complex pediatric interventional procedures

Cath labs are predominantly staffed by a interdisciplinary team composed of registered nurses, cardiovascular technologists, and radiology technologists as well as clerical and support staff, depending on the department's size. How roles and responsibilities are delineated can be very different among hospitals, regions, states, and countries. Staff working in the cath lab should maintain Advanced Cardiac Life Support certification, and if pediatric procedures are done, Pediatric Advanced Life Support certification.

All cath labs have their own unique cultures. Working in the cath lab requires an attitude of continual learning, a commitment to teamwork, and effective communication skills. When involved in procedures and patient care, meticulous attention to detail is needed. You work more closely with physicians than in the typical nursing unit setting. Busy or high volume cath labs are dynamic areas with rapidly changing schedules, add-on cases, and emergencies. Staff cannot do a procedure by themselves—it takes a team of skilled inter-disciplinary staff to assist and provide care to increasingly complex patients during increasingly complex procedures.

TEAMWORK IN THE CATH LAB

Teamwork is essential, as no one staff member can assist with a procedure without others doing their part. Important components of effective teamwork include:

- Shared goals
- Active listening and communication
- Conflict resolution skills
- Adaptability and flexibility
- Diversity of skill sets
- Effective leadership

During procedures, it is common to have a minimum of three team members who assist the cardiologist: the scrub assistant, the circulating assistant, and the monitoring/recording assistant. Some complex procedures may require additional staffing support. Each role is uniquely important to the completion of procedures and registered nurses can be trained for each role.

CATH LAB STAFF ROLES

Scrub Role

The scrub assistant:

- Sets up the sterile table, including the manifold (if used), and pressure and injector tubings and flushes catheters
- Wears a sterile gown and gloves and stands next to the physician at the x-ray table to assist with access, sheath placement, and guidewire/catheter manipulation
- Prepares medications on the table, for example, lidocaine, heparin, and nitroglycerin
- Injects contrast and medications from the sterile table

Circulating Role

The circulator:

- Reviews the patient's medical record
- Assists the patient to the table

- Applies various monitors, including the cardiac monitor, noninvasive blood pressure monitor, pulse oximetry, and end-tidal carbon dioxide ($ETCO_2$) monitor
- Administers procedural sedation and other medications as ordered by the physician
- Monitors and assesses the patient's responses during the procedure
- Obtains equipment and supplies from within the procedure room
- Documents in the patient's medical record

Monitoring Role

The monitor/recording staff member:

- Obtains needed equipment and supplies
- Assists the patient to the table, applying and initiating monitoring
- Ensures high-quality electrocardiographic tracings are obtained
- Records hemodynamic waveforms and enters pressure measurements into the physiological monitor during the procedure
- Ensures the accuracy of the data used for various calculations
- Completes various reports needed for the physician and the patient's medical record

ABOUT CARDIOVASCULAR TECHNOLOGISTS

Cardiovascular technologists commonly work within the cath lab setting. They are often graduates from a 1- to 2-year cardiovascular program where they are taught in great detail about hemodynamics and learn to scrub and monitor. In some states, they may be allowed to administer medications under the physician's direct supervision.

ABOUT RADIOLOGY TECHNOLOGISTS

Radiology technologists work in cath labs and often operate the x-ray equipment. Many are trained to scrub and monitor. In some states, they may be allowed to administer medications.

They are responsible for:

- Oversight of the x-ray equipment, including quality assurance
- Moving the x-ray table (panning) during the procedure
- Making x-ray system changes as needed

Often a radiology technologist oversees the cath lab radiation safety program, ensuring personal dosimeter monitoring badges are worn by all staff and physicians and are regularly replaced, and posts the exposure reports.

WORKING IN A SURGICAL ENVIRONMENT

Procedures are completed using sterile technique to decrease the risk of infection to the patient. You will need to learn sterile technique and how to correctly maintain and work within the sterile field. A controversial change over the past several years has been the trend toward requiring cath labs to adopt and follow operating room standards for all procedures, not just open surgical procedures like pacemaker and implantable cardioverter–defibrillator implantation. This shift is being driven by regulatory agencies such as the Centers for Medicare & Medicaid Services and The Joint Commission.

Your cath lab may be required to maintain the same environmental standards as the operating room, including identification of restricted and semirestricted spaces, air exchanges, and specific room temperature and humidity guidelines.

Cath lab staff may be expected to adhere to surgical attire guidelines and:

- Wear hospital-laundered surgical scrubs
- Cover their head/hair with single-use bouffant hats and cover facial hair
- Cover their mouth/nose with disposable surgical masks during procedures

Essential Facts

- Prepare your sterile table as close to the time of use as possible.
- Wear a sterile gown, cap, mask, and gloves when setting up the table/tray.
- Look for tears in packaging before opening an item for the sterile field.
- Check sterility indicators to confirm sterilization has occurred.
- Keep your hands and arms above the waist.
- Pass sterile items to the sterile field in a way that maintains sterility.

(continued)

(continued)

- Do not allow nonsterile items to come in contact with the sterile field.
- Do not pass a nonsterile item over the sterile field.
- Do not lean over the sterile field if you are not scrubbed in.
- Do not pass between two sterile fields if you are not scrubbed in.
- Do not eat or drink in the procedure rooms.

Surgical Scrub

Prior to scrubbing in on a procedure, a surgical hand and forearm scrub is performed as follows:

- Remove rings and watch.
- Use a nail pick to clean under nails.
- Scrub fingertips, fingers, and hands on all sides with a scrub brush impregnated with chlorhexidine or povidone-iodine.
- Wash forearms on all sides up to just below the elbows with the sponge side of a scrub brush.
- Scrub should last at least 2 minutes.
- Rinse each hand and arm with the hand held upward so that water runs down the arms.

Waterless scrub solution is also available for use with subsequent scrubs and should be applied per the manufacturer's recommendations.

Donning Sterile Attire

After scrubbing, the following applies:

- Keep hands upward when entering the procedure room.
- Take a sterile towel from the table and pat dry your hands from fingertips to forearms.
- Don the sterile gown, without touching the outside of the gown; another staff member will adjust the back of the gown and tie it up.
- The front of the sterile gown is considered sterile from the chest to the level of the sterile field (the table or the draped patient).
- The parts of the gown considered unsterile include the neckline, shoulders, underarms, and back.
- Keep the cuff of the sterile gown covered by the glove.

There are two techniques for donning sterile gloves: the closed method and the open method. Identify which technique is preferred in your new setting. Wear two pairs of sterile gloves when scrubbing to decrease the risk of blood exposure.

Sterile Table Setup

The basic supplies and equipment needed for table setup and patient preparation often come bundled together in a large sterile pack:

- The outer nonsterile protective covering is removed and the pack is placed on the table.
- The outer wrap of the pack becomes the table drape as it is unfolded and opened.
- Only the top surface of a sterile draped table is considered sterile; the edges and sides are considered nonsterile even though they are covered by the drape.

Sterile table setup varies; become familiar with the way it is done in your cath lab. If staff set their tables similarly, the easier it is to relieve for breaks or lunch.

SUMMARY

Various procedures are done in the cath lab setting and increasingly more complex procedures that once required open surgery are now done using catheter-based technologies in cath lab procedure rooms and hybrid labs. An interdisciplinary team, led by the cardiologist, is essential in safely completing these procedures. It is important to understand everyone's role and contribution to the procedure. To learn more about working in a surgical environment, refer to *Essentials for the Operating Room Nurse* or review the most recent edition of Association of periOperative Registered Nurses' (AORN) *Guidelines for Perioperative Practice*.

2

Working in an X-Ray Environment

The use of x-ray is required in order for cath lab procedures to be completed. Physicians use fluoroscopy for placing and advancing sheaths, guidewires, catheters, balloons, stents, and other devices. Angiographic images are acquired during cath procedures and become a part of the patient's medical record. Nurses are typically not educated about working in an x-ray environment. This chapter provides an overview of x-ray and working safely in the cath lab.

In this chapter, you will learn:

1. Cath lab x-ray equipment, including the gantry, digital image detector, and x-ray table
2. Differences between fluoroscopy, image acquisition, and digital subtraction angiography (DSA)
3. Stochastic and deterministic effects of radiation
4. Ways to reduce occupation radiation exposure

CATH LAB X-RAY EQUIPMENT

The most dominant feature in a cath lab procedure room is the C-arm and x-ray table (Figure 2.1).

- The gantry holds the x-ray tube and the image detector across from one another
- The gantry may be ceiling mounted or floor mounted

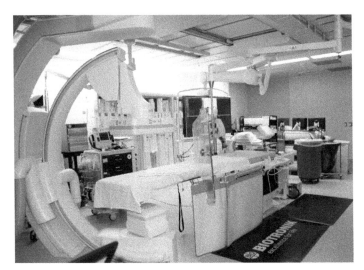

Figure 2.1 Cath lab C-arm.

- The patient lies on the x-ray table and the gantry moves around the patient.
- The gantry rotates in two directions: right/left and cranial/caudal.

The x-ray tube is where the x-ray beam, or direct beam, is created. It is mounted on the lower part of the gantry. The x-ray beam travels in a straight line through the patient to the image detector on the opposite side where the x-ray is converted into an image. Digital image detectors have now widely replaced the image intensifier (II) that was used before digital technology was available; however, you may still hear the image detector referred to as the II.

Cath lab x-ray systems operate in three modes:

- Fluoroscopy is also referred to as *fluoro*. It is used for real-time continuous imaging for guidewire and catheter placement; it is activated when needed via a foot pedal controlled by the cardiologist or the radiologic technologist.
- Image acquisition is the digital recording of high-quality angiographic images; you may sometimes hear it referred to as cine, short for cineangiography, which is an older term used when images were recorded on film rather than digitally acquired.
- DSA is used for imaging noncardiac stationary vessels, like the carotid or the iliac arteries. DSA delivers a higher dose of radiation. In this mode, the overlying bone and soft tissue are removed, or subtracted, from the image, leaving only the vessels showing.

The cardiologist or the radiology technologist uses the tableside controls to adjust the gantry movement around the patient, the field of view, and the magnification mode. Moving the table or *panning* during image acquisition is often needed to see the entire structure or course of the artery. Many physicians do their own panning, but this is not always the case.

Essential Facts

Check your hospital policies and procedures to see if you are able to move the patient on the table while the x-ray is being generated. Regulations vary among states, but in many areas, only the physician and x-ray technologists are permitted to do this.

POTENTIAL HEALTH RISKS OF X-RAYS

Exposure to radiation has the potential to harm cells and tissues. Radiation exposure is cumulative and its effects are permanent. These effects are described as *stochastic* or *deterministic*.

- Stochastic: It damages cellular DNA, which increases with increasing total radiation dose. Examples of stochastic effects include genetic alterations, brain tumors, and leukemia.
- Deterministic: The effect is predictable and dose-dependent and risk increases as the radiation dose increases. Examples of deterministic effects include cataracts and skin pigment changes, burns, and hair loss on the patient at the x-ray entrance site.

MINIMIZING X-RAY EXPOSURE TO THE PATIENT

All procedures should be necessary, justified, and completed with the goal of keeping radiation exposure as low as reasonably achievable (ALARA). Efforts taken to minimize x-ray exposure to the patient also minimize exposure to the cardiologist and the staff.

Essential Facts

To reduce x-ray exposure to the patient, follow these guidelines:

- Use the lowest acceptable fluoroscopy dose and frame rate.
- Use pulsed fluoroscopy.

(continued)

(*continued*)

- Use "fluoro save" or "fluoro store" option.
- Limit magnification.
- Use collimators whenever possible.
- Keep the II/image detector as close to the patient as possible.
- Keep the table as high as comfortable.
- Vary angulation of the imaging beam as possible to minimize repetitive exposure to one site on the patient.
- Minimize the use of prolonged steeply angled views whenever possible.
- Keep the patient's extremities out of the direct beam.

Scatter Radiation

As the x-ray beam travels through the patient, some of the x-ray is bounced off the patient, or redirected, in all directions. This redirected secondary x-ray is referred to as scatter radiation.

Essential Facts

Scatter radiation is the primary source of staff exposure to radiation when working in an x-ray environment. Most scatter will travel in the direction of the image detector.

Three key things to remember in protecting yourself from x-ray exposure include:

- Time
- Distance
- Shielding

Time

Use x-rays only when imaging is needed. Reducing the duration of x-ray exposure will reduce the dose.

Distance

The farther you are from the x-ray source, the less exposure you will receive. Doubling your distance from the x-ray source will reduce radiation exposure by a factor of 4. This is the inverse square law and it states that the intensity of radiation decreases in proportion to the square of the distance from the source. When you are scrubbing, step back behind the operator during image acquisition if possible. When circulating, stand/sit behind a moveable shield when not providing direct patient care.

Shielding

Lead aprons are protective apparel made of vinyl impregnated with lead, tin, and other metals to attenuate the scatter. Aprons are available in different thicknesses of shielding, ranging from 0.25 to 1 mm lead equivalent (LE). A 0.5 mm LE apron provides greater than 90% shielding from scatter. Aprons should be readily available in multiple sizes. Many facilities provide custom lead aprons for staff.

Different types of aprons are available, such as front protection, one-piece wraparounds, or two-piece vest and skirt sets. Wraparound aprons are recommended for maximum protection. When fitting lead aprons, the goal is to cover the torso from the neck to the knee to protect the long bones of the legs. Use of poorly fitting lead aprons can lead to unnecessary radiation exposure. Large armholes can allow scatter to the breast tissue. Thyroid collars should also be worn as the thyroid is sensitive to radiation. When the thyroid collar is on, there should be no gaps between the thyroid collar and the neck of the apron.

When not in use, hang lead aprons on designated racks designed to hold their weight. To prevent cracking, aprons should not be folded during storage. Assess lead aprons and thyroid collars at least once per year for defects, such as cracking or holes, that could allow radiation to pass through. If defects are noted, the piece should be removed from use, sent for repair if possible, or replaced with a new piece.

- Use the hanging radiation protection shield during procedures. When correctly positioned, it blocks up to 90% of scatter to the operator's head and neck.
- Wear 0.25 mm leaded glasses with side shields to protect the lens of the eye when scrubbed in. Cataracts are a documented risk of chronic radiation exposure.
- Consider wearing lead caps when scrubbed in. Progress is being made with producing lighter weight caps that can reduce radiation to the head by 80%.
- Use lead table skirts. The physician and scrub person receive the most exposure from below the table during a procedure because of the proximity of the x-ray tube and x-ray tube leakage.
- Use disposable radiation absorbing towels and drapes if possible.

The consistent use of moveable shields, lead glasses, thyroid collars, lead aprons, and table skirts substantially reduces your exposure to scatter x-ray.

MONITORING EXPOSURE

Personal radiation monitors are worn by staff working in x-ray areas to measure occupational exposure. Three types of monitors are available: film badges, thermoluminescent dosimeters, and optically stimulated luminescent dosimeters. The badges do not provide real-time exposure reporting; they measure cumulative exposure. They are monitored periodically and reports should be posted. The inconsistent use of personal dosimeters leads to underestimation of radiation exposure. Real-time dosimeters are also available for use. See Table 2.1 for more information on personal dosimeters.

Occupational Limits

Occupational dose limits (DL) have been established by the National Council on Radiation Protection and Measurements (NCRP). NCRP recommends a maximum effective DL of 50 mSv/y with a cumulative lifetime DL of 10 mSv multiplied by age for radiation workers. Exposure to 1 milligray (mG) of radiation produces a dose of 1 mSv. Additionally, recommendations are in place for DL for the lens of the eye and parts of the body.

- DL for lens of eye: 150 mSv/y
- DL for extremities: 500 mSv/y
- DL for embryo-fetus: 0.5 mSV/mon

Table 2.1

Dosimeter Use

- Wear dosimeters while at work. Always! Wear at neck/collar level outside of your lead apron/thyroid collar to approximate eye and thyroid exposure.
- Some hospitals may require the use of two dosimeters: one outside of the lead apron and one underneath it. Do not get them mixed up!
- Do not leave personal dosimeters in procedure rooms when you are not assisting with the procedure.
- Know where to locate and how to interpret the report of your personal readings.
- Do not keep film badges in an enclosed vehicle where temperatures can become very high.

Life-time occupational exposure is monitored. When moving to another facility, request that your records be transferred.

Pregnant Workers

If a cath lab team member chooses to declare her pregnancy, she should meet with the radiation safety officer to better understand safe working standards. She should be given a second real-time dosimetry device to wear at the waistline under lead shielding. The monthly equivalent dose to the fetus should not exceed 0.5 mSV and the limit for the entire pregnancy should not exceed 5.0 mSV, according to the Nuclear Regulatory Commission.

Procedural Monitoring

During procedures, the patient's exposure to x-ray is monitored. Depending on your x-ray system, methods for doing this include the following:

- Fluoroscopy time is expressed in minutes and it is the total time fluoroscopy is used during the procedure. It does not include image acquisition (cine) time. It is the least useful measure of x-ray exposure.
- Air Kerma (AK) is expressed in grays, or Gy. It is the cumulative dose of x-ray exposure delivered during a procedure at a specific defined reference point. It is closely associated with deterministic skin effects.
- Dose area product (DAP) is expressed in $Gycm^2$. It is the total amount of radiation delivered to the patient including both fluoroscopy and image acquisition (cine) time. It estimates the stochastic risks to the patient.

Patients can develop early transient erythema of the skin with 2 Gy of direct radiation exposure. The physician should be notified if 3 Gy is reached. Each 1 Gy after that should be called out and documented in the patient's medical record. Patients who receive high levels of exposure need to be taught to monitor their backs for skin redness or irritation and to call the procedural physician if skin changes are noted. Permanent skin discoloration and ulceration can occur as a result of exposure.

Essential Facts

- Patients receiving substantial radiation exposure (>5 Gy) should be counseled before hospital discharge and receive appropriate follow-up.

(continued)

(*continued*)

- If a patient receives greater than 10 Gy of x-ray exposure, a medical physicist should be consulted to calculate peak skin dose.
- The Joint Commission considers exposures over 15 Gy in a single procedure a reportable sentinel event.

Hospitals typically have a radiation safety committee and/or a radiation safety officer who has oversight over all departments using radiation. Learn as much as you can about working in an x-ray area to help promote radiation protection awareness and education in your cath lab.

Regulatory agencies responsible for radiation protection standards include the NCRP, the U.S. Environmental Protection Agency, the Food and Drug Administration, and the Occupational Safety and Health Administration.

SUMMARY

Working in an x-ray environment is new for many nurses coming in to the cath lab. It is important to have a basic understanding of how the x-ray equipment works and how to protect yourself from scatter radiation through time, distance, and shielding. A major goal of a successful procedure is to obtain good imaging, while ensuring the patient's exposure is minimized as much as possible.

3

About Contrast Media

Contrast media (CM) contain iodine, which absorbs x-rays and makes the images black. The iodine concentration required for coronary angiography ranges from 300 to 370 mg/mL. Contrast media are categorized by osmolality and ionicity. Osmolality is the concentration of a solution, expressed as the total number of solute particles per kilogram of solution, while ionicity indicates if it is ionic or nonionic.

In this chapter, you will learn:

1. About different types of CM
2. Who is at most risk for contrast reactions
3. How to manage contrast reactions
4. How to identify the patient at risk of acute kidney injury (AKI) following contrast administration
5. Strategies to decrease the risk of AKI

TYPES OF CM

The use of CM is required in most procedures done in the cath lab. CM used in today's cath labs are low or iso-osmolar and nonionic. See Table 3.1 for additional information on currently used contrast agents. Rarely used in today's cath lab are the high-osmolar ionic contrasts such as diatrizoate (Renografin, Hypaque) and Iothalamate

Table 3.1

Types of Contrast	
	Generic/Brand Name
Low osmolar, nonionic	Iopamidol (Isovue), iohexol (Omnipaque), ioversol (Optiray), ioxilan (Oxilan)
Iso-osmolar, nonionic	Iodixanol (Visipaque)

(Conray). These contrasts commonly caused significant bradycardia and hypotension.

All patients should be screened for contrast allergies prior to procedure. Contrast may be administered by the cardiologist or by staff via an automated injector, a handheld manifold, or a syringe. Key points to keep in mind about the administration of contrast:

- Patients may feel a warm sensation, especially in the pelvic region, during contrast injection of the left ventricle.
- Transient bradycardia, hypotension, nausea, and/or vomiting can occur following contrast administration.
- Contrast can damage kidneys; the smallest amount possible should be administered.
- Document the total volume of CM administered in the patient's medical record.

CONTRAST REACTIONS

Patients can have a hypersensitivity or anaphylactoid reaction to contrast that is non–immunoglobulin E mediated. It is thought that the contrast activates the mast cells and basophils, causing a release of histamine.

Risk Factors for Contrast Reaction

Patients with a previous contrast reaction have the highest risk of developing a recurrent reaction. A previous reaction increases patients' overall risk fivefold. Other at-risk patients include those with a history of:

- Asthma, bronchospasm, or atopy
- Other severe drug and/or food allergies
- Concurrent beta-blockers or metformin

Essential Facts

A common misperception is that patients with an allergy to shellfish are also allergic to contrast. When patients have an allergic reaction to seafood, they are reacting to a specific muscle protein (tropomyosins and parvalbumin) within the seafood, not the iodine.

Mild contrast reactions typically include sneezing, flushing, itching (pruritus), and/or an urticarial rash. They are usually self-limiting and can be quickly and effectively treated with diphenhydramine 25 mg to 50 mg IV.

More serious contrast reactions can include:

- Angioedema
- Laryngospasm and bronchospasm
- Stridor, wheezing, and respiratory distress
- Hypotension
- Tachycardia

Treatment of serious reactions includes:

- Stopping further contrast administration
- Giving epinephrine 0.3 mL 1:1,000 dilution SC or IM, or 3 mL 1:10,000 dilution IV
- Starting supplemental oxygen, if not already in place; assess airway as intubation may be needed
- Giving aggressive fluid resuscitation with normal saline (NS) or lactated Ringer's boluses for hypotension
- Giving additional medications, including diphenhydramine 50 mg IV, methylprednisolone 80 mg to 125 mg IV, and/or ranitidine 50 mg IV or cimetidine 300 mg IV; for sustained respiratory distress and hypotension, an epinephrine infusion may be started at a rate of 2 mcg/kg/min to 20 mcg/kg/min, depending on the severity of the symptoms and the patient's response

Delayed reactions to contrast can occur up to a week following its administration. Signs and symptoms may include:

- Skin rash
- Fever
- Fatigue
- Abdominal pain
- Joint pain

Pretreatment of Known Contrast Allergy

In patients who have previously experienced a contrast reaction, pretreatment with corticosteroids and histamine blockers is indicated. It is important to understand that pretreatment may not prevent all contrast reactions. Commonly used pretreatment protocols include the following:

- For elective procedures: Prednisone 50 mg PO at 13, 7, and 1 hour prior to the procedure plus diphenhydramine 50 mg PO 1 hour prior to the procedure
- For urgent/emergent procedures: Methylprednisolone sodium succinate 40 mg IV or hydrocortisone sodium succinate 200 mg IV every 4 hours until the administration of contrast and diphenhydramine 50 mg IV 1 hour prior to contrast administration

CONTRAST-INDUCED ACUTE KIDNEY INJURY

CM is potentially nephrotoxic and can cause worsening of renal function. Contrast-induced acute kidney injury (CI-AKI) has been defined as deterioration of renal function following the administration of contrast in the absence of other causes or a rise in serum creatinine of greater than 0.5 mg/dL (or a 25% increase from baseline) within 48 to 72 hours of contrast administration that cannot be attributed to other causes.

It is the third-leading cause of hospital-acquired AKI; CI-AKI affects 5% to 40% of patients who receive contrast. Risk factors for developing CI-AKI are outlined in Table 3.2. It generally peaks within 3 to 5 days with gradual resolution within 2 to 3 weeks.

Table 3.2

Risk Factors for CI-AKI	
Pre-existing renal insufficiency (eGFR <60 mL/min/1.73 m^2)	Hypotension
Contrast load exceeding 3.7 mL × eGFR	Heart failure
	EF <40%
	Anemia
Diabetes	Chronic use of NSAIDs
Advanced age	Concurrent nephrotoxic medications
Female gender	Peripheral arterial disease
Dehydration	

CI-AKI, contrast-induced acute kidney injury; eGFR, estimated glomerular filtration rate; EF, ejection fraction; NSAIDs, nonsteroidal anti-inflammatory drugs.

While short-term dialysis may be needed in a small number of patients, permanent renal failure from CI-AKI is rare.

The most powerful predictor for developing CI-AKI is the presence of pre-existing chronic kidney disease. Evaluating the patient's serum creatinine level is not the best assessment. Glomerular filtration rate (GFR), or the amount of blood that passes through the glomeruli per minute, provides a more accurate assessment of nephron function. An estimated GFR (eGFR) can be derived from the serum creatinine level, adjusted for variables such as age, sex, weight, nutritional status, and race. Normal eGFR is greater than 60 mL/min/1.73 m^2.

Essential Facts

A patient with an eGFR less than 60 mL/min/1.73 m^2 may be at increased risk for CI-AKI.

Many hospitalized patients receive multiple doses of contrast from various imaging procedures they may have. Normal kidneys take about 20 hours to clear contrast. The staging, or spacing out, of non-urgent procedures is an important consideration to prevent CI-AKI. In preparing for elective procedures, it is beneficial to hold potentially nephrotoxic drugs such as nonsteroidal anti-inflammatory agents, aminoglycosides, and antifungals for 24 hours for patients at risk of CI-AKI. Metformin (Glucophage) is an oral diabetic agent that has been associated with severe and potentially fatal lactic acidosis when contrast is administered in patients with renal insufficiency. It should be held for 48 hours and the patient's serum creatinine should be reassessed before it is restarted.

Several risk stratification tools have been developed and can be found in the literature. It may be standard in your cath lab to calculate the maximal acceptable contrast dose (MACD) as a guideline for upper limits of contrast administration. See Table 3.3 for one common method of determining MACD. Keep in mind that some patients will develop CI-AKI with volumes of contrast lower than

Table 3.3

Calculating Maximal Acceptable Contrast Dose (MACD)
Formula: 3.7 × eGFR = upper limit of contrast dose in mL.
Example: Your patient's eGFR is 86 mL/min/1.73 m^2.
MACD = 86 × 3.7 = 318.2 mL contrast

eGFR, estimated glomerular filtration rate.

their calculated MACD. It is important to use the least required amount of contrast for adequate visualization. Staff should notify the cardiologist when approaching the upper limits of MACD. The cardiologist may choose to continue the procedure and administer additional contrast, but it remains your responsibility to notify them when MACD is reached and to document in the patient's medical record.

HYDRATION STRATEGIES TO DECREASE CI-AKI

Hydration has been found to be the most beneficial approach in decreasing the incidence of CI-AKI and should be considered prior to the procedure. Examples include the following:

- Normal saline (NS) 0.9% or 0.45% NS 1 mL/kg/hr is given for 6 to 12 hours prior to contrast administration and continued for 6 to 24 hours following the procedure. The patient should be monitored closely for signs of fluid overload.
- NS boluses may be administered based on the measured left ventricular end-diastolic pressure (LVEDP); for example, 3 mL/kg/hr for LVEDP of 13 mmHg to 18 mmHg or 5 mL/kg/hr for LVEDP greater than 13 mmHg.
- Oral hydration has also be found to be helpful and should be encouraged following procedures if the patient is able to take fluids.

PHARMACEUTICAL STRATEGIES TO DECREASE CI-AKI

Ascorbic acid may be useful for some patients. Statins may provide benefit through their antioxidant and anti-inflammatory effects. Additional research is needed to substantiate the possible benefits of ascorbic acid and statins.

Medications that have been evaluated and been found to be ineffective for decreasing the risk of CI-AKI include:

- Acetylcysteine
- Bicarbonate
- Dopamine
- Fenoldopam
- Furosemide
- Mannitol
- Theophylline

SUMMARY

For the nurse new to the cath lab, it is important to learn about CM. Contrast administration should be monitored closely. Some patients will have reactions to contrast that can range from hives to full cardiovascular collapse. Know how to support your patient during a contrast reaction. Learn to identify and treat those patients at risk of developing CI-AKI.

4

Procedural Patient Preparation

Before a planned procedure is started, there are many things you need to do to be fully prepared. The procedure room needs to be checked to ensure all needed equipment and supplies, including emergency items, are readily available. The patient's medical record should be carefully reviewed. Introduce yourself to the patient and let the patient know your role. Be reassuring and work to build rapport with the patient and the family, if present. Answer their questions as clearly and professionally as possible.

In this chapter, you will learn:

1. Components of procedure room setup
2. Key preprocedure assessment findings
3. Points for patient preparation
4. Which patients are at risk with moderate sedation
5. Essential elements of the universal protocol
6. Medications commonly used for procedural sedation

CHECKING THE PROCEDURE ROOM

Most cath labs have a system of checking the procedure rooms before bringing patients into the room. This is done to ensure that emergency equipment and supplies are readily available in the room and in good working order. Checklists can be helpful so that items are not overlooked. The defibrillator in the room is assessed according to the manufacturer's recommendations to ensure it charges and paces appropriately. Airway supplies, oxygen, and cannulas and masks should be easily obtainable. Suction should be checked. Other equipment that should be readily available include infusion pumps, a temporary pacemaker generator with a pacing wire, an intra-aortic balloon pump and/or Impella console.

GETTING TO KNOW YOUR PATIENT

Patient Identification

Prior to bringing patients into the procedure room, always identify them using two patient identifiers. Many facilities routinely use the patient's name and date of birth or medical record number.

History and Physical

The patient's documented history and physical (H&P) needs to be current (within 30 days of procedure) with a focused update done within 24 hours of procedure. Review the H&P, including indications for the planned procedure. Look to see if the patient has undergone cardiac stress testing or previous cardiac procedures such as percutaneous coronary intervention (PCI) or coronary artery bypass graft (CABG) surgery. If they've had previous PCI or CABG, see if you can find what coronary arteries were ballooned, stented, or bypassed. Note relevant comorbidities such as:

- Diabetes
- Peripheral arterial disease
- Renal insufficiency
- Severe hypertension
- Valvular heart disease
- Advanced pulmonary disease

Essential Facts

Check Blood Pressure in Both Arms
On arrival to the prep area, assess blood pressure (BP) in both arms. A systolic pressure difference of 10 mmHg or more suggests subclavian artery disease. Angiography of the left internal mammary artery may be needed if coronary artery bypass surgery is indicated.

Allergies

Always ask the patient if they have any allergies and determine the type of reaction they experienced. Allergies to contrast, heparin, aspirin, latex, or metals can impact the procedure that is planned and are especially important to note. Patients with previous contrast allergies should be premedicated with steroids and antihistamines and this is reviewed in detail in Chapter 3.

Nil per Os (NPO) Status

It is common practice to restrict the patient's oral intake prior to procedures by keeping them *nil per os* (NPO) to decrease the risk of aspiration in case of nausea and vomiting during the procedure. Some hospitals may allow patients to have clear liquids up to the time of the procedure. Be familiar with your hospital's policies and procedures about NPO status and sedation/anesthesia administration.

Current Medications

Carefully review all medications the patient is currently taking, including over-the-counter medications, vitamins, and herbal supplements. Some herbal supplements can increase the risk of bleeding, including feverfew, garlic, ginger, ginkgo biloba, and St. John's wort.

- Warfarin is usually stopped 3 days before elective invasive procedures when femoral access or device implantation is planned.
- Diuretics are generally held the day of the procedure to decrease risk of dehydration.
- Oral hypoglycemic agents are often held the day of the procedure.
- Half-dose insulin is often given the day of the procedure, accounting for the length of time the patient will be NPO.
- Metformin and all combination medications containing metformin should be held on the day of the procedure and for 48 hours afterward.
- Erectile dysfunction medications should be held for 24 hours before elective procedures.

Preprocedure Diagnostic Testing

Prior to planned procedures, most patients have additional diagnostic testing done. Some common tests that may be done include:

- Noninvasive stress testing, including exercise, stress echocardiography, or nuclear medicine myocardial perfusion imaging.

- Twelve-lead EKG to assess for arrhythmias, bundle branch blocks, and ST segment changes.
- Pregnancy test for females of childbearing age.
- Complete blood count (CBC) to assess for anemia and thrombocytopenia.
- Serum creatinine to obtain estimated glomerular filtration rate (eGFR).
- Coagulation testing for patients who routinely take warfarin; the international normalized ratio (INR) goal is less than 1.8 to decrease the risk of bleeding when femoral artery access is planned.
- Type and screening or crossmatch may be done for complex or high-risk procedures where there is an increased risk of hemorrhage and the need for transfusion.
- Chest x-ray may be indicated if the patient has clinical signs and symptoms of heart failure with volume overload.

Informed Consent

Informed consent is a legal process that ensures patients have been told by their physician of the risks, benefits, and alternatives to the procedure as well as possible outcomes and potential complications that may occur. At many hospitals, an emergent patient with ST-segment elevation myocardial infarction (STEMI) activation may be an exception for the informed consent process. Review your own hospital's policies and procedures.

- The physician should explain the procedure to the patient, in the patient's native language, and in terms the patient can easily understand.
- The patient must be competent.
- Informed consent should be provided in neutral setting, not the procedure room.
- The patient's signature may be required on a legal document verifying he or she received informed consent.

Preprocedure Sedation

Some physicians may order oral antianxiolytic agents be given prior to taking the patient into the procedure room. Examples of common oral preoperative agents include diazepam, lorazepam, and diphenhydramine.

Airway Assessment Prior to Procedural Moderate or Deep Sedation

Medications such as IV midazolam and fentanyl are often used for sedation during the procedure. See Table 4.1 for more information

Table 4.1

	Medications for Procedural Sedation	
	Typical Initial Dosing	**Nursing Implications**
Opioids		
Fentanyl	25–50 mcg IV. MR as needed every 5 minutes. Short half-life. More potent than morphine.	■ All opioid analgesics/ sedatives can cause respiratory depression, hypoventilation, and hypercapnia.
Morphine	2–4 mg IV. MR every 5–30 minutes as needed.	■ Monitor respiratory rate, oxygen saturation, and capnography levels.
Hydromorphone (Dilaudid)	0.5–1 mg IV	■ Know your hospital's conscious sedation/ procedural sedation policies and procedures.
Meperidine (Demerol)	25–50 mg IV	
Benzodiazepines		
Midazolam (Versed)	0.5–1 mg IV. MR every 5 minutes as needed.	■ Benzodiazepines provide anxiolytics and induce a hypnotic state, amnesia, and sedation.
Diazepam (Valium)	5–10 mg PO for preprocedure anxiety. 2.5–5 mg IV slowly (burns at injection site).	■ They do not have analgesic properties.
Lorazepam (Ativan)	0.25–1 mg IV	■ They can cause respiratory depression and hypotension at higher doses.
		■ Lorazepam has a slower onset of action and longer duration (6–8 hours) than midazolam and diazepam.
Other		
Diphenhydramine (Benadryl)	25–50 mg IV	■ Use with care in asthma.
Reversal Agents		
Naloxone (Narcan)	0.4–2 mg IV every 2–3 minutes PRN to increase respiratory rate and level of consciousness.	■ To reverse oversedation with narcotics such as fentanyl, morphine, and/or hydromorphone.
		■ Monitor for resedation due to naloxone's short half-life.

(continued)

Table 4.1

Medications for Procedural Sedation (*continued*)

	Typical Initial Dosing	Nursing Implications
Flumazenil (Romazicon)	0.2 mg IV every 1 minute PRN to max dose of 3 mg/hr.	■ To reverse oversedation with benzodiazepines such as midazolam, diazepam, or lorazepam. ■ Monitor for resedation due to flumazenil's short half-life.

IV, intravenous; MR, modified repeat.

Table 4.2

American Society of Anesthesiologists (ASA) Physical Status Classification System

1—Patient is healthy; has no systemic disease

2—Patient has mild systemic disease; no functional limitations

3—Patient has severe systemic disease

4—Patient has severe systemic disease that is a constant threat to life

5—Patient is not expected to survive without the procedure

6—Patient has been declared brain-dead; organs are being removed for donor purposes

Source: Adapted from American Society of Anesthesiologists (ASA). (2014). Retrieved from https://www.asahq.org/resources/clinical-information/asa-physical-status-classification-system

about agents commonly used for procedural sedation. Moderate sedation is adequate for many cath procedures while deep sedation or general anesthesia may be indicated for more complex procedures.

The patient should be assessed by the physician prior to receiving IV sedation and narcotic agents. The American Society of Anesthesiologists (ASA) Physical Status Classification System is commonly used by the physician to describe the patient's risk. See Table 4.2 for details.

Specific airway assessment is required prior to the administration of sedation and/or general anesthesia. The Mallampati Score is a tool developed to assess the ease of intubation or a physical exam to ensure the patient can easily open the mouth fully, lift the chin, and move the neck. See Table 4.3 for additional details. Patients who are unable to open the mouth fully or rotate the neck easily can be difficult to intubate if needed.

Table 4.3

Mallampati Score	
Class I	The complete soft palate can be visualized with the mouth open. Intubation is usually easy.
Class II	The uvula can be visualized with the mouth open. Intubation is usually easy.
Class III	Only the base of the uvula can be visualized with the mouth open. Intubation may be moderately difficult.
Class IV	The soft palate is not visible at all with the mouth open. Intubation may be very difficult.

Source: Adapted from Naidu, S. S., Aronow, H. D., Box, L. C., Duffy, P. L., Kolansky, D. M., Kupfer, J. M., . . . Blankenship, J. C. (2016). SCAI expert consensus statement: Best practices in the cardiac catheterization laboratory. *Catheterization and Cardiovascular Interventions.* doi:10.1002/ccd.26551. Retrieved from www.scai.org

Key points to remember about procedural sedation:

- Procedural sedation is ordered by the physician and administered by the nurse or technologist, depending on hospital policy and state law.
- Patient factors that can lead to problems with procedural sedation include obstructive sleep apnea or a history of snoring, obesity, and a short neck or limited range of motion of the neck.
- Required monitoring during procedural sedation includes oxygen saturation, end-tidal carbon dioxide ($ETCO_2$), BP, respiratory rate, and cardiac rhythm and rate at frequent intervals.
- If you administer procedural sedation, you need to be familiar with airway management techniques and use of a bag-valve-mask device in the event you need to rescue the patient.
- Reversal agents including naloxone and flumazenil need to be readily available.

Pulses

The presence, amplitude, and symmetry of pulses should be assessed prior to the procedure. Commonly assessed pulses include bilateral femoral, pedal, posterior tibial, and radial pulses. A commonly used grading scale to describe pulses is a 0 to +4 scale.

- 0 = absent pulse
- +1 = diminished or decreased pulse
- +2 = normal

- +3 = full pulse
- +4 = bounding pulse

Procedure Room

After all the prep work is completed, the patient can then be moved into the cath lab procedure room and placed in a supine position on the x-ray table. Several monitoring devices are attached and include:

- Cardiac monitor: An optimal electrocardiographic monitor is essential during procedures, especially when performing coronary intervention. Before starting the procedure, assess the cardiac rhythm, rate, and ST segments. Most hemodynamic monitoring systems include a five-lead system that displays multiple leads on the monitor. Radiolucent electrodes and leads are available. Place the electrodes and the cables so that they do not interfere with the movement of the gantry.
- Noninvasive BP monitor: Place the cuff on the nonintravenous arm (whenever possible) and begin recording intermittent BP readings.
- Oxygen saturation monitor: This assesses the adequacy of oxygenation. Monitor the SpO_2 continuously. Normal SpO_2 is 95% to 100%. Remember that an SpO_2 of 90% roughly equals an oxygen saturation of 60 mmHg on an arterial blood gas.
- $ETCO_2$ monitor: This assesses the adequacy of ventilation. It measures exhaled CO_2 and helps assess for hypoventilation and CO_2 retention. Normal $ETCO_2$ is 35 mmHg to 45 mmHg.

Defibrillator

A defibrillator is required in very close proximity to the patient during the procedure so that you are able to rapidly defibrillate when needed. Place defibrillation pads on patients at high risk for arrhythmias; for example, patients experiencing a STEMI. In many cath labs, defibrillation pads may be routinely placed on all patients.

Patient Prep

Know the planned access site and prep accordingly. Most cath labs prepare bilateral groin sites for a planned femoral approach and the wrist and a femoral site for a radial approach. Skin preparation at the access site is important. The goals of skin preparation include the following:

- Remove hair using clippers as needed for draping.
- Clipping of body hair should occur outside of the procedure room to decrease the risk of contamination.

■ Remove debris, exudate, and microorganisms from the skin to decrease the risk of infection.

For obese patients with a large pannus, pulling the pannus up superiorly and taping it can help in locating the optimal site for arterial access. Palpate the groin to assess location of the maximal femoral pulse.

Commonly used prep solutions include 2% chlorohexidine and 70% isopropyl alcohol (Chloraprep, Becton Dickinson) or povidone-iodine (Betadine). Apply per the manufacturer's recommendations. In some labs, the skin prep may be done by the scrub assistant or it may be done by the circulator. For a moist area such as the groin, prep for 2 minutes. It is essential to allow the prep solution to dry for 3 minutes before draping the patient. Avoid pooling of the prep solution as this can be a fire hazard.

Patient Draping

A sterile drape with bilateral femoral openings, or fenestrations, is used to create the sterile field on the patient after the prep is completed and the prep solution has dried. If a radial approach is planned, an additional sterile drape is placed over the arm.

If a break in sterile technique is recognized, corrective action should be taken as quickly as possible. This may include removing contaminated instruments or supplies, changing gloves, redraping with new sterile drapes, and/or administering an antibiotic.

Antibiotic Prophylaxis

The administration of an antibiotic prophylaxis is not typically indicated for most cath lab procedures but should be considered when a device will be implanted, as with pacemakers and implantable cardioverter defibrillators, valve repair/implantation, and defect closures.

Universal Protocol

The universal protocol, or procedural time-out, is a safety measure to ensure that the correct procedure is being done on the correct patient. Site marking may not needed for cath lab procedures as the heart can be approached from several areas. Key elements of the universal protocol include:

■ Confirming the correct patient
■ Confirming the planned procedure
■ Ensuring needed equipment, supplies, devices, and implants are readily available

While the universal protocol is being performed, all team members should pause in their activities and actively participate in the process as much as possible without compromising patient safety.

SUMMARY

Thorough room and patient preparations are essential for a smooth procedure. All essential equipment and supplies should be in good working order and readily available. As a nurse in the procedure room, it is your responsibility to know the patient's history and current diagnostic findings. To ensure patient safety, when the patient is brought into the room, make certain that the appropriate monitors are placed; sedation, if ordered, is given according to accepted guidelines; and the universal protocol is completed correctly.

5

Arterial Access

One of the most important parts of a cath procedure is obtaining the arterial access that is needed for catheter placement. The most common complications of cath procedures are related to bleeding and hematoma development at the puncture site. The cardiologist's goal is to be able to puncture the artery and the vein perfectly on the first attempt. Cath lab staff play an important role in the early recognition and management of vascular complications.

In this chapter, you will learn:

1. Local anesthetics commonly used
2. Femoral and radial artery access
3. Equipment needed for obtaining arterial access
4. Complications of arterial access

LOCAL ANESTHESIA

Local anesthetics produce numbness by reversibly inhibiting excitation of nerve ending or by blocking conduction in peripheral nerves. They primarily block the sensation of sharp pain, though patients will still feel pressure when the sheath is placed or removed.

Lidocaine (Xylocaine)

- Lidocaine is most commonly used for cath lab procedures.
- Different concentrations are available, including 1%, 2%, and 4%. Higher concentrations of lidocaine increase the risk of toxicity and do not shorten the onset of action or prolong local anesthesia.
- Its onset is within 2 minutes to 5 minutes and effects last up to 60 minutes.
- Dose should not exceed 4 mg/kg or a maximum of 300 mg (30 mL of a 1% solution or 15 mL of a 2% solution).
- The pH of lidocaine is acidotic (pH 5–7). This can cause burning with subcutaneous (SC) injection. To counter this, lidocaine can be buffered with sodium bicarbonate. One milliliter of sodium bicarbonate of a 1 mEq/mL solution can be added to every 9 mL of lidocaine.
- For patients allergic to lidocaine, procaine (novocaine) can be used. Its onset of action is 5 minutes to 10 minutes and effects last up to 90 minutes.
- Diphenhydramine can also be used for local anesthesia.

Bupivacaine (Marcaine)

- Bupivacaine may be used in pacemaker or device placements or for procedures expected to be lengthy.
- Different concentrations are available, including 0.25% and 0.5% concentrations. Bupivacaine 0.25% should be used for local infiltration if the patient is awake as the 0.5% concentration is painful when injected.
- Its onset of action is within 10 minutes and effects last up to 4 hours.
- It should not be buffered as precipitation can occur.

Local anesthetic should be administered slowly SC, often starting with a 25-gauge needle and then changing to a 21- or 22-gauge needle to infiltrate a deeper and wider area. You'll see the physician aspirate prior to injecting, looking for blood return that would indicate the needle is within a vessel.

There are two types of reactions to local anesthesia: an immediate urticaria and anaphylaxis or a delayed dermatitis characterized by swelling, rash, and blistering. Toxicity from local anesthesia is uncommon but can be seen. If toxicity is suspected, stop the procedure, resuscitate as indicated, protect airway, control muscle tremors/seizure with diazepam, and treat bradycardia with atropine.

Signs and symptoms that indicate neurotoxicity include:

- Lightheadedness, tinnitus, double vision, seizures
- Circumoral numbness, metallic taste

- Mental status changes, slurred speech
- Bradycardia, hypotension

MODIFIED SELDINGER TECHNIQUE

The modified Seldinger technique is commonly used for vascular access. After the local anesthetic is injected, puncture of the artery or vein is done, a guidewire is placed through the needle, and the needle is then removed. The sheath with the dilator in it is placed over the guidewire and advanced into position. The guidewire is then removed. The side arm of the sheath is aspirated and flushed.

EQUIPMENT NEEDED FOR VASCULAR ACCESS

Equipment needed for successful vascular access includes:

- Local anesthetic of choice
- Needles, syringes, and saline
- Micropuncture kits
- Guidewire and sheath
- Ultrasound

Needles

For femoral access, commonly used needles include an 18- or 19-gauge thin-wall open-bore needle with a bevel tip or a Seldinger-type needle that contains a stylet. Both are about 3 inches (7.62 cm) in length and accommodate a 0.035 inch (0.09 cm) guidewire.

A micropuncture kit may be used for radial, brachial, and femoral access. The kit comes with a 21-gauge needle, a 0.018 inch (0.05 cm) steerable floppy-tipped guidewire, and a 4 Fr sheath. Using fluoroscopy, the 0.018 inch (0.05 cm) guidewire is advanced under fluoroscopic guidance through the micropuncture needle. Angiography is done via the 4 Fr sheath to confirm that the puncture site is in the appropriate location. The 4 Fr sheath is then exchanged for a 0.035 inch (0.09 cm) guidewire and the appropriately sized sheath is placed over the guidewire.

Guidewires

The size of guidewire used most commonly when obtaining femoral access is 0.035 inch (0.09 cm). Short guidewires come in the sheath kit. Standard guidewires are 145 cm to 150 cm length; they are also readily available in 300 cm, which is needed for exchanging catheters. Guidewires are made of stainless steel (most common), nitinol, and/or platinum with an inner core wire that can be fixed or moveable. They are usually tapered with a flexible atraumatic tip, which can be straight or curved. Factors that differentiate guidewires include wire length, tip length, wire stiffness, and the coating.

Sheaths

Sheath kits contain the sheath with a side arm, a dilator, and a short guidewire; sizes from 4 Fr through 7 Fr are commonly used. Sheath length can range from 11 cm to 35 cm or more depending on the manufacturer. Longer sheaths are useful when the patient is found to have significant arterial tortuosity. The hub of the sheath contains a one-way valve designed to prevent back-bleeding. The side arm allows for flushing, blood sampling, pressure measurement, or contrast injection.

Ultrasound

The use of ultrasound to guide access is increasing. It can be very helpful when pulses are faint or not palpable. With ultrasound, the needle, the femoral artery, and the bifurcation can all be easily visualized, helping to decrease the risk of an arterial puncture that is too high or too low or the unintentional puncture of the femoral vein. Heavy calcification can also be seen. The use of ultrasound guidance reduces the number of attempts, reduces time to access, reduces accidental venous puncture, and decreases vascular complications. Needles with an ultrasound transducer at the tip are also commercially available.

FEMORAL ARTERY ACCESS

Anatomy Review

- The common femoral artery (CFA) is a continuation of the external iliac artery at the level of the inguinal ligament. The CFA is a large vessel and is not prone to spasm.
- The CFA then branches into the superficial femoral artery (SFA) and the profunda femoris (or deep femoral) artery.
- The femoral vein lies just medial to the femoral artery.
- The femoral nerve lies lateral to the femoral artery.

Femoral access remains the most commonly used approach for cath procedures in the United States but the radial approach is increasing in popularity. Retrograde (against flow) sheath placement in the CFA is the most common sheath placement. The optimal puncture for femoral artery access is a single front-wall puncture at the midpoint of the CFA over the center of the femoral head. The puncture should be below the inguinal ligament and above the bifurcation of the CFA.

External landmarks such as the skin/inguinal crease are not accurate in identifying the location of the CFA. It can be especially difficult in some patients who have diminished femoral pulses, are obese, or have extensive scarring from previous procedures.

Using fluoroscopy, visualize the bony landmarks such as the femoral head. The tip of a metal hemostat can be placed at the inferior border of the femoral head to use as a guide. The cardiologist can then puncture the skin at a 45° angle to enter the CFA just below the center line of the femoral head. With the puncture over the femoral head, compression is easier when the sheath is removed.

Femoral angiography is the gold standard to assess the CFA arteriotomy site. To perform this technique, inject contrast through the side arm of the sheath after the sheath is in place. This provides information about the location of the arteriotomy in relationship to the bifurcation as well as vessel size (Figure 5.1).

Vascular complications can be directly related to the quality of the femoral arterial puncture. Key points to remember:

- The femoral artery angiography should be taken at an ipsilateral 20° to 30° (right anterior oblique [RAO] for right CFA puncture, left anterior oblique [LAO] for left CFA puncture) rather than a straight anteroposterior view. This provides better visualization of the CFA bifurcation into the SFA and the deep femoral artery.
- Femoral artery angiography should always be done prior to the deployment of a vascular closure device (VCD).

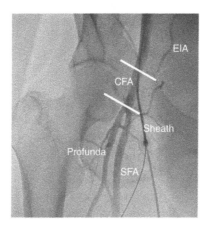

Figure 5.1 Femoral angiography.
CFA, common femoral artery; EIA, external iliac artery; SFA, superficial femoral artery.

- High sticks, above the origin of the inferior epigastric artery into the external iliac artery, increase the risk of retroperitoneal hemorrhage (RPH).
- Low sticks are associated with increased incidences of hematomas, vessel laceration, pseudoaneurysms (PSAs), and arteriovenous (AV) fistulas because of inadvertent placement of the sheath into the SFA or the smaller profunda femoris artery. Additionally, low punctures are made below the femoral head, making compression more challenging because there is no bone to compress against.

Antegrade Femoral Artery Sheath Placement

In antegrade sheath placement, the sheath is placed with its distal tip toward the foot rather than up toward the abdomen. It is much less commonly performed than retrograde puncture. It is more technically challenging compared with retrograde puncture. It can be challenging to do in obese patients. Antegrade sheath placement is indicated for below-the-knee interventions. A sharper angle of entry is required to avoid puncturing the external iliac artery. The sheath entry may be higher. Bleeding, hematoma, and vascular injury are more common with antegrade puncture.

RADIAL ARTERY ACCESS

Anatomy Review

- The radial artery originates from the brachial artery below the elbow and runs on the lateral aspect of the forearm to the wrist, where it lies on top of the styloid process of the radius bone and the schapoid bone.
- The artery then joins the deep communicating branch of the ulnar artery to form the deep palmar arch.

The radial approach has several advantages over femoral access. The radial artery is easily compressed and bleeding complications are uncommon. It can be especially helpful for patients with severe peripheral arterial disease or for those with morbid obesity. The hand has collateral flow from the ulnar artery via the palmar arch. Prolonged bed rest is not required so patients are able to be up and about soon after the procedure is complete.

Left radial access is beneficial in the patient who has a left internal mammary artery (LIMA) graft to the left anterior descending (LAD) artery. It is easier to cannulate the LIMA from the left radial than from the right radial artery.

For cardiologists who are accustomed to doing femoral punctures only, obtaining radial access can be technically challenging and there can be a steep learning curve. During the learning process, there may be longer case times and increased radiation exposure, but that improves as experience and confidence are gained. In many centers now, radial is the preferred approach.

Allen's Test

Prior to performing radial artery puncture, the Allen's test is performed to assess ulnar flow to ensure the palmar arch is intact and collateral flow is present.

- Simultaneously occlude the radial and the ulnar arteries while having the patient make a fist.
- Ask the patient to then open the hand. The palm of the hand will appear pale and blanched.
- Release pressure over the ulnar artery. If pink color returns to the palm within 6 to 10 seconds, it is a positive result, meaning there is satisfactory ulnar flow and radial access can be safely performed.
- The test is considered negative or abnormal if it takes more than 10 seconds for the palm to be pink.

Assessment of ulnar flow can also be done using a pulse oximetry with plethysmography. The pulse oximeter probe is placed on the ipsilateral thumb or forefinger and the radial and ulnar arteries are compressed. The waveform will flatten. Then remove pressure from the ulnar artery, keeping pressure on the radial. In a normal test, the waveform will return. The test is considered abnormal if the waveform does not return or if there is a delay of more than 8 seconds in return of color to the hand.

Contraindications to Radial Access

- Lack of radial pulse
- Raynaud's disease

Patient Prep for Radial Access

The patient's IV should be placed in the opposite arm. The patient should be comfortably sedated to decrease anxiety.

The patient's arm is moved away from the body at an angle. The wrist is then positioned and hyperextended while supported with a small towel or roll of gauze. There are also commercially available positioning devices.

The radial area is prepped and draped. A small amount of local anesthetic (1–2 mL) is infiltrated using a 25-gauge needle. The ideal puncture site is 2 cm to 3 cm proximal to the flexor crease of the wrist. The use of ultrasound may be helpful. A through-and-through or double-wall puncture is preferred for the radial artery. A micropuncture needle kit may be used for a single-wall puncture with the 21-gauge needle, 4 Fr or 5 Fr catheter, and 0.018 inch (0.05 cm) guidewire. A hydrophilic sheath is advanced over the guidewire into the radial artery.

Before a catheter is advanced through the radial sheath, it is common to administer a "cocktail" through the sheath side arm to decrease the risk of radial artery spasm. The drugs used in the intra-arterial (IA) cocktail varies and includes some combination of heparin, verapamil, diltiazem, nitroglycerin, nicardipine, lidocaine, nitroprusside, and/or adenosine. The cocktail can be mixed with blood and administered over a minute to decrease patient discomfort. Anticoagulation is needed in radial access because of the risk of thrombosis. Heparin, which is what causes the discomfort, may also be given separately by IV injection.

When advancing the guidewire, stop if any resistance is felt. There may be an arterial loop or an accessory artery present. It may be helpful to perform angiography to further define the anatomy.

Essential Facts

Left radial access may be preferred if angiography of the LIMA is needed.

For more information on radial access, go to the website at http://www.transradialuniversity.com.

BRACHIAL ARTERY ACCESS

Anatomy Review

- The brachial artery is a continuation of the axillary artery.
- It runs to the medial side of the antecubital fossa and divides into the radial and the ulnar arteries.

Historically, cath procedures for brachial access were accomplished by a surgical cutdown known as the Sones technique. Today, percutaneous techniques are used for sheath placement in the right brachial artery. The brachial artery may be chosen for access for an obese patient or when femoral access cannot be obtained.

Patient Prep for Brachial Access

The arm is abducted, an armboard is placed, and the site is prepped and draped. Percutaneous access is obtained using a thin-wall needle or a micropuncture kit may be used. Anterior wall puncture is preferred. A vasodilator "cocktail" may also be used with brachial access to decrease the risk of arterial spasm. Anticoagulation is needed in brachial access because of the risk of thrombosis.

For sheath removal, manual pressure is most commonly used to obtain hemostasis. VCDs have been used in brachial access but it is an off-label use. Brachial artery access is associated with a higher complication rate.

VASCULAR COMPLICATIONS

Femoral Artery Access Complications

Vascular complications, including bleeding, hematoma formation, pseudoaneurysm (PSA), RPH, AV fistula, and limb ischemia are the most common complications following cath lab procedures, occurring in about 6% of patients. Factors that contribute to this include anticoagulation/antiplatelet therapy, larger sheath sizes, and female gender. Major postcath bleeding and blood administration are associated with a longer length of stay and decreased long-term survival rates.

Hematoma

A hematoma is a collection of blood in the anterior compartment of the thigh and is the most common vascular complication following cath lab procedures. The incidence of hematoma following cath procedures is less than 5%. A large hematoma can cause compression of the femoral nerve, causing limb weakness and paresthesia, or can lead to deep vein thrombosis.

- Risk factors for hematoma development include ineffective compression, failure of a VCD, obesity, hypertension, advanced age, female gender, and aortic insufficiency.
- Treatment includes manual compression and fluid boluses as needed; blood transfusions may be indicated.
- An expanding hematoma, despite pressure, should prompt a vascular surgery; consult for possible open surgical repair and evacuation.

Pseudoaneurysm

A PSA is an abnormal or false continued communication between the femoral artery and the hematoma. The incidence of PSA is reported to be less than 1% following coronary interventional procedures. A PSA can cause neuropathy by compressing adjacent structures and can be a nidus for infection. Interestingly, left femoral access has been associated with an increased risk of PSA.

- Risk factors for PSA development include low arterial puncture of the SFA or profunda artery, inadequate manual or mechanical compression, or excessive anticoagulation.
- Signs and symptoms include a painful, very tender-to-touch groin. A pulsatile mass can be palpated and a bruit is heard when auscultated with a stethoscope.
- The presence of a PSA is confirmed by Doppler ultrasound imaging.
- Treatment is indicated if the PSA diameter is greater than 3 cm, using ultrasound-guided thrombin injection (500–10,000 IU) into the neck of the PSA. Surgical repair may be indicated for a large PSA.

Retroperitoneal Hemorrhage

RPH occurs when there is free bleeding into the retroperitoneal space, which can hold large volumes of blood. It is the most serious and potentially lethal complication of femoral arterial access. The incidence of RPH is less than 1% of procedures performed from the femoral artery.

- Risk factors include a high femoral puncture or posterior wall puncture, full anticoagulation, and the concurrent use of IIb/IIIa glycoprotein inhibitors. Other risk factors include female gender, chronic renal insufficiency, and low body weight.
- Signs and symptoms can be subtle and include unexplained hypotension, tachycardia, pallor, and back, flank, or lower quadrant abdominal pain. Bleeding into the retroperitoneal cavity stimulates the vagal nerve and symptoms of increased vagal tone can be seen, including bradycardia, nausea, diaphoresis, and pallor.
- A CT scan is done to confirm the diagnosis.
- Treatment needs to be prompt and aggressive. Anticoagulation should be stopped if possible. Serial hematocrits should be done. Normal saline boluses and blood products may be administered to maintain volume. Vasopressor agents may be needed in addition to fluid boluses. Placement of a covered stent, balloon tamponade, or open surgical repair may be indicated if the patient continues to be hypotensive with dropping hematocrits.

AV Fistula

An AV fistula forms when both the femoral artery and the femoral vein are punctured and a persistent connection between the two is formed. It is an uncommon complication with a reported incidence of less than 1%.

- Risk factors include low femoral puncture or the inadvertent puncture of a vein while accessing the artery.
- Signs and symptoms include pain. A thrill can be palpated and a bruit can be auscultated.
- An AV fistula is confirmed by Doppler ultrasound imaging.
- Treatment is generally open surgical repair.

Arterial Thrombosis

Thrombosis of the femoral artery is an uncommon complication.

Essential Facts

Signs and symptoms of arterial thrombosis include the six Ps in the affected leg: pain, paresthesia, pallor, pulselessness, paralysis, and/ or poikilothermia (temperature changes).

- Risk factors include small caliber vessel, peripheral arterial disease, and large sheath size.
- A vascular surgeon is often consulted and treatment may include heparin, thrombolytic therapy, thrombectomy, or open surgical repair.

Infection

Infection at the femoral artery access site is uncommon but can cause significant morbidity. The reported incidence is less than 0.05%. Persistent hematoma can be a nidus for infection.

- Risk factors include obesity, diabetes, compromised sterile technique, prolonged sheath dwelling time, repeat procedure at same site, and use of a VCD.
- Signs and symptoms include manifestation of redness and tenderness, drainage, fever, and elevated WBC.
- Treatment includes antibiotics and comfort measures. Surgical intervention may be needed, especially if the infection is due to a VCD.

Arterial Dissection

Femoral artery dissection is an uncommon complication. Most patients are asymptomatic and most dissections heal.

RADIAL ARTERY ACCESS COMPLICATIONS

Complications and access site bleeding rates are much lower in radial access than in femoral access. With the growth in radial approach, complications unique to the radial artery have been identified.

Radial Artery Spasm

Spasm is a common complication of radial catheterization, occurring in up to 20% of cases. Causes include inadequate sedation, repeat access attempts, and catheter exchanges. Spasm can lead to difficulty accessing the artery, advancing and removing catheters, and can lead to catheter entrapment. To prevent entrapment, an antispasm cocktail is commonly administered after access is obtained. Rarely, a patient may require additional sedation to manage radial artery spasm.

Radial Artery Occlusion

The incidence of radial artery occlusion may be as high as 10%. It results from endothelial vessel injury and subsequent neointimal hyperplasia, thrombosis, and external mechanical compression of the vessel. Risk factors include high sheath-to-artery ratio, occlusive hemostasis rather than patent hemostasis, and lack of anticoagulation use. Radial artery occlusion limits future radial access and limits the use of the radial artery for dialysis or as a conduit for bypass grafts. Patients may not have symptoms but those who are symptomatic may need surgical intervention.

Radial Artery Perforation

Perforation of the radial artery can be caused by forceful manipulation of the sheath, wire, or catheter. Bleeding into the soft tissue with hematoma formation can occur at the site of the sheath insertion or along the course of the artery. Risk factors for perforation include radial loops and tortuosity. Forearm hematoma can occur with perforation. A large hematoma can cause hand ischemia and pain. Compression with an inflated blood pressure cuff may be indicated.

Compartment Syndrome

Compartment syndrome can develop with an expanding hematoma in the forearm, leading to nerve and muscle damage. Suspect this in the postprocedure patient who is experiencing the six Ps: pain, paresthesia, pallor, pulselessness, paralysis, and/or poikilothermia (temperature changes).

Compartment syndrome is a rare but serious complication. Urgent fasciotomy is indicated.

Pseudoaneurysm

PSA of the radial artery is very rare. Risk factors include multiple punctures, use of large sheaths, and poor positioning of the compression device, or ineffective compression. Patients develop pain and swelling at the puncture site. It is diagnosed by color Doppler ultrasound and is treated with ultrasound-guided thrombin injection.

Radial Artery Avulsion

Radial artery avulsion is caused by intense spasm during sheath removal. For patients having spasm, treat aggressively with vasodilators, additional sedation/analgesia, and slowly remove the sheath. If unable to remove, general anesthesia may be needed.

Sterile Granuloma

The hydrophilic coating on the access sheath can cause chronic inflammation, leading to the formation of a sterile granuloma at the puncture site in some patients. An ultrasound should be done to rule out a PSA. Treatment for a sterile granuloma is surgical drainage.

BRACHIAL ARTERY ACCESS COMPLICATIONS

- Hematoma, thrombosis, PSA
- Damage to the median nerve
- Compartment syndrome

SUMMARY

Obtaining arterial access is an important part of the procedure that can be associated with complications. For femoral access, the optimal puncture site is the CFA. Complications may occur with a sub-optimal femoral puncture. Radial access is growing in popularity and there are fewer complications associated with the radial approach but they can still occur.

6

Hemostasis and Vascular Closure Devices

Hemostasis is controlling the bleeding by the formation of a platelet plug and a fibrin mesh that develops the clot. The ability to obtain hemostasis readily is essential to decrease bleeding and vascular complications following cath lab procedures. Sheath removal should be done as soon as safely possible following the procedures to decrease the risk of bleeding and vascular complications. Increasingly, vascular closure devices (VCDs) are being used.

In this chapter, you will learn:

1. Factors important to know when removing femoral sheaths
2. Applying manual pressure correctly
3. Available adjuncts for mechanical pressure
4. Differences among the available VCDs
5. Tips for radial sheath removal

There are several factors to consider when removing femoral arterial sheaths, including:

- Sheath size
- The patient's anticoagulation status
- Blood pressure

HEMOSTASIS WITH FEMORAL ACCESS

Many facilities use point-of-care testing with activated clotting time (ACT) or clinical lab testing with activated partial thromboplastin time (aPTT) to guide the timing of sheath pulling. For example, the cardiologist may indicate that the sheath is to be removed when the ACT is less than 180 seconds or the aPTT less than 45 seconds. Other facilities may designate a time for the sheath to be pulled. For example, the cardiologist may indicate that the sheath is to be removed in 4 hours.

When it is time to remove the sheath(s), assess the patient's vital signs and ensure they are free of chest pain, check to ensure you have an IV that flows well as the patient may need a fluid bolus, and allow the patient to empty the bladder if needed. Some cardiologists may order a small amount of narcotic for comfort.

Essential Facts

It can be difficult to obtain hemostasis in the patient with marked hypertension. Prior to sheath removal, or early in the hemostasis period, it can be very helpful to obtain an order for and administer a short-acting antihypertensive medication, such as hydralazine or metoprolol.

A decision that you will need to make is the choice of using manual or mechanical pressure, or it may be ordered by the physician. Position the height of the bed or gurney for your comfort. You want to be able to comfortably apply manual pressure rapidly if needed. Manual pressure can be fatiguing. If the patient has both an arterial and a venous sheath in the same side, remove the arterial sheath first, get hemostasis of the arterial site, and then remove the venous sheath.

Manual Pressure

Manual pressure is considered the gold standard for obtaining hemostasis. Pressure is applied in a steady and controlled manner, using two or three fingers centered 2 cm above the arterial entry site, and as the sheath is removed, apply firm and constant pressure. During manual pressure, the distal pedal and/or posterior tibial pulses should not be completely obliterated. A faint distal pulse should remain palpable to ensure some distal blood flow.

Time frames for holding pressure can vary, depending on sheath size and the amount of anticoagulation administered, but a period of 15 minutes to 30 minutes is usually needed. If bleeding recurs, manual pressure should be quickly reapplied. Some hospitals may use an algorithm based on sheath size; for example, for an arterial sheath, 3 minutes of manual pressure per French size. Thus, with a 6 Fr sheath, the minimal hold time would be 18 minutes.

Mechanical Pressure

One of the earliest devices developed for mechanical pressure is a C-clamp device. It has a flat metal plate that is placed under the patient's hip. An adjustable arm holds a sterile disk that is placed over the puncture site. Pressure is applied as the arm is lowered and locked into place. Other smaller handheld compression devices are also available.

The Femostop (St. Jude Medical, Inc.) is a commonly used mechanical device that uses pneumatic compression to apply pressure over the femoral arterial puncture site. A hard plastic frame, held in place with a strap around the patient, holds a transparent inflatable dome. The dome is positioned slightly superior to the access site, and as the sheath is removed, the dome is inflated with a hand pump to a pressure slightly higher than the patient's blood pressure.

The Safeguard (Merit Medical) device is a combination sterile dressing/pressure balloon that is inflated over the site as the sheath is removed.

VASCULAR CLOSURE DEVICES

The use of VCDs has dramatically increased in recent years; they reduce time to hemostasis, facilitate patient mobilization, and decrease hospital length of stay. There are multiple VCDs on the market that have been designed to obtain immediate hemostasis at the end of the procedure.

Femoral artery angiography should be performed prior to the deployment of a VCD to ensure that the puncture site is clearly identified. Prior to the placement of a VCD, it is recommended that the deployer change to new sterile gloves and reprep the access site and arterial sheath to decrease the risk of infection.

VCDs can be divided into two categories based on how they work:

- One type deploys a suture or clip at the arteriotomy and examples include ProStar XL, Perclose ProGlide, and StarClose SE (Abbott Medical).
- Another type deploys an absorbable plug, sealant, or gel at/ over the arteriotomy site. Examples include Angio-Seal (St. Jude Medical, Inc.), VASCADE (Cardiva Medical, Inc.), and the Mynx (Cardinal Health).

Contraindications to the use of VCDs include:

■ Multiple arterial punctures.
■ Suboptimal arteriotomy site, such as a puncture in the superficial femoral artery (SFA) or the profunda femoris (deep femoral) artery. They also should not be used if the puncture is above the internal iliac artery or at the bifurcation.
■ Placement in synthetic grafts or through a femoral stent is not recommended.

The overall complication rate of VCD use is about 2%. Infection following deployment of a VCD is an uncommon but serious complication. Groin infections require aggressive medical management and possible open surgery. Infections are associated with severe morbidity, prolonged hospitalization, prolonged antibiotic use, and increased mortality.

Some centers allow cath lab staff to deploy VCDs. Typically there is a required portion of didactic education and return demonstration to ensure staff are fully competent with the device. It is important that staff also be able to recognize when it is not appropriate to deploy, for example, with a suboptimal arteriotomy site. Know your hospital's policies and procedures about this.

Preclosure Technique for Large Arterial Sheaths

Preclosure technique is used to close large arteriotomies needed for procedures requiring large (>12–24 Fr) sheaths. This technique preloads a suture around the puncture site prior to placement of large arterial sheaths. Two ProGlide devices are placed across from each other and the sutures are placed before the initial dilation of the artery and then the arteriotomy can be closed with the two sutures when the procedure is completed. This is off-label use.

HEMOSTASIS PADS

Pads or patches that facilitate hemostasis are available. They contain substances such as D-glucosamine, calcium alginate, or polyprolate acetate that promote local clot formation. Examples include Neptune Pad (TZ Medical), Clo-Sur P.A.D. (Merit Medical), and StatSeal (Biolife LLC).

HEMOSTASIS WITH RADIAL ARTERY ACCESS

The radial sheath should be removed as quickly as possible at the end of the procedure. Before removal, flush the sheath. Verapamil or nitroglycerin may again be given intra-arterially. The sheath is removed as manual pressure or mechanical pressure with a bracelet-type band is applied using the concept of patent hemostasis. Several different radial compression devices are commercially available, including TR Band (Terumo Interventional Systems), HemoBand, and TRAcelet (Medtronic).

Patent Hemostasis

Patent hemostasis is applying enough pressure to stop the bleeding but not enough to completely occlude the vessel and stop all distal flow. It has been found to decrease the rate of radial artery occlusion. To do this, perform the following:

- Withdraw the arterial sheath 2 cm to 3 cm and apply the compression device over the skin entry site.
- Remove the sheath and tighten the device firmly.
- Then begin to decrease the pressure in the device until mild pulsatile bleeding at the skin entry site is seen.
- After two or three cycles of pulsatile bleeding, retighten the device just enough to stop the pulsatile bleeding.

Maintain the arm and wrist in a neutral position for patient comfort. The patient is able to be up and about as tolerated. Monitor for bleeding, swelling, skin color changes, capillary refill, and discomfort. Compression should be maintained for 60 minutes to 120 minutes with gradual release of pressure occurring during this time period.

HEMOSTASIS WITH BRACHIAL ARTERY ACCESS

Manual compression is recommended when removing brachial arterial sheaths, as control of bleeding can be more difficult with this approach. Some cardiologists may choose to deploy a VCD; however, this is off-label use.

KEY POINTS FOR PATIENT CARE FOLLOWING SHEATH REMOVAL

Femoral Approach

- After hemostasis is obtained, clean the site and apply a small dressing. A large dressing can hide a hematoma.
- Visually assess the site frequently. Gently palpate for potential hematoma formation.
- If bleeding or hematoma development occurs, reapply manual pressure.

- Follow your cardiologist's orders or hospital policy for bed rest. In general, bed rest is recommended for 2 hours to 6 hours, depending on the size of the arterial sheath and whether a VCD was used.
- The patient's head of bed may be elevated up to 30 degrees.
- Sandbags over the puncture site have been found to be ineffective in preventing bleeding/hematoma formation.
- Patient teaching points: Do not your lift head up off the bed/ gurney. Hold your groin site for coughing/sneezing and so on. Keep the affected leg flat. Call for help if you feel something warm or wet in the groin.
- Prior to discharge, palpate for a pulsatile mass and auscultate for a bruit. These findings suggest a pseudoaneurysm may be present.

Essential Facts

Vigilant nursing assessment is essential when caring for patients immediately following femoral artery sheath removal. The fibrin clot can be dislodged and the patient can bleed extensively in a short period of time. The site should be visualized and palpated frequently. This is also important in patients who received a VCD as late failure can occur.

Radial Approach

- After hemostasis is obtained and the radial band is removed, clean the site and apply a small dressing.
- Visually assess the site frequently. Gently palpate for potential hematoma formation.
- If bleeding or hematoma development occurs, reapply manual pressure.
- Follow your cardiologist's orders or hospital policy for bed rest. In general, bed rest is not required following removal of a radial sheath.
- Patient teaching points: Do not use the affected hand/arm for 24 hours; gradually increase your activities.

SUMMARY

Obtaining stable hemostasis following removal of access sheaths is essential, regardless of the access site. Close patient monitoring for bleeding, hematoma formation, or other potential vascular complications is imperative. Early intervention by cath lab staff can make a big difference in patient outcomes.

7

Cath Lab Hemodynamics: Waveforms, Pressures, and Calculations to Know

Hemodynamics is the interrelationship of pressure, flow, and resistance within the cardiovascular system. When working in the cath lab, it is essential that you have a thorough understanding of hemodynamics. During diagnostic cardiac catheterization, pressure measurements from various chambers of the right and left heart are obtained and recorded. Fick and thermodilution cardiac output (CO) can be determined. These data are then used by the hemodynamic system to calculate multiple parameters such as aortic and mitral valve areas and shunt calculations.

In this chapter, you will learn:

1. Factors that affect accuracy in monitoring
2. Normal heart pressures and normal oximetry findings
3. Reasons for abnormalities in waveforms, pressures, and oximetry findings
4. Techniques for measuring CO
5. Measuring shunts and calculating aortic and mitral valve areas

ACCURACY IN MONITORING

Obtaining accurate hemodynamic profiles requires accuracy in monitoring, leveling, and data entry. Common causes of inaccuracy that can lead to errors in pressure measurements include:

- Improperly leveled or zeroed transducers
- Air bubbles, thrombus, or kinks in the pressure tubings
- Damaged transducer
- Loose connections
- Artifact—overdamping, overshoot, catheter fling

The transducer should be level with the midchest at the phlebostatic axis, which is the landmark on the chest where the midchest line intersects the fourth intercostal space. It represents the anatomic position of the atrium. If the transducer is too high, or above the phlebostatic axis, the pressure will be artificially low; conversely, if the transducer is too low, or below the phlebostatic axis, the pressure will be artificially high.

RIGHT HEART WAVEFORMS, PRESSURES, AND CALCULATIONS

About the Right Atrial Waveform and Pressure

The right atrium (RA) receives blood from the superior vena cava (SVC) and the inferior vena cava (IVC). The RA waveform consists of positive and negative waves referred to as A and V waves and X and Y descents (Figure 7.1). In the RA, the A wave is larger than the V wave. The mean RA pressure is the average of the waves. Normal mean RA pressure is 1 mmHg to 8 mmHg. Normal breathing and changes in intrathoracic pressures affect the RA and left atrium (LA), so pressures should be measured at end expiration. The normal oxygen saturation range for the RA is 70% ± 5%.

- A wave: It represents RA contraction with the peak just after the P wave on the ECG. In the RA position, the A wave is larger than the V wave. An A wave is not present in atrial fibrillation, atrial flutter, and some junctional rhythms.
- X descent: It follows the A wave and indicates the drop in RA pressure.
- C wave: It is not always seen. It represents closure of the tricuspid valve.
- V wave: It represents passive filling of the RA. The peak of the V wave corresponds to the opening of the tricuspid valve.
- Y descent: It follows the V wave and represents passive emptying of the RA.

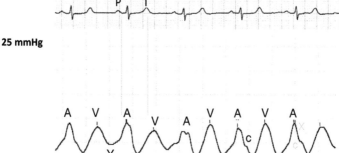

X descent
and V upslope
=systolic events

V peak, Y, and A
=diastolic events

Figure 7.1 Atrial pressure tracing with A-X-V-Y. Note the timing of the peak of the V wave with respect to the end of the electrocardiographic T wave, and A wave with respect to the P wave. The C wave is a small positive deflection on the atrial tracing that sometimes interrupts the X descent and corresponds to the brief protrusion of the tricuspid valve into the RA in early systole during isovolumic ventricular contraction. The C wave splits X into a segment that corresponds to atrial relaxation (X) and another segment that corresponds to annular descent (X').

RA, right atrium.

Source: From Hanna, E. B., & Glancy, D. L. (2013). *Practical cardiovascular hemodynamics with self-assessment problems.* New York, NY: Demos Medical Publishing, LLC.

Abnormalities in the RA waveform and pressure readings can be caused by the following:

- Low RA pressure will be seen in hypovolemia.
- Prominent A waves will be seen in tricuspid stenosis, right ventricular hypertrophy, right heart failure, cardiac tamponade, and complete heart block.
- Prominent V waves will be seen in right heart failure and tricuspid regurgitation.
- Deep X and Y descents will be seen in constrictive pericarditis and restrictive cardiomyopathy.

About the Right Ventricular Waveform and Pressure

As the catheter is advanced from the RA through the tricuspid valve to the right ventricle (RV), an abrupt change in the waveform morphology will be seen. The waveform will appear more rectangular.

The waveform has a sharp upstroke, which corresponds to the contraction, or systole, of the RV. It is recorded as a phasic pressure—systolic and end-diastolic pressures. Normal RV pressures are 15 mmHg to 30 mmHg systolic and 2 mmHg to 7 mmHg diastolic. The normal oxygen saturation range for the RV is 70% ± 5%.

Essential Facts

The right ventricular end-diastolic pressure (RVEDP) is an indicator of overall health of the RV.

Abnormalities in the RV waveform and pressure readings can be caused by the following:

- Low RV pressure will be seen in hypovolemia.
- Elevated end-diastolic pressure will be seen in RV failure.
- Elevated systolic pressures will be seen in pulmonary hypertension and pulmonary embolism.
- A "dip and plateau" pattern (Figure 7.2) can be seen in RV failure, constrictive pericarditis, and restrictive cardiomyopathy.

About the Pulmonary Artery Waveform and Pressure

The catheter is advanced from the RV through the pulmonic valve to the pulmonary artery (PA). The waveform appearance changes again and becomes more triangular looking as the catheter is advanced from the RV into the PA. The dicrotic notch correlates to the closure of the pulmonic valve. It is recorded as a phasic pressure (systolic, diastolic) and mean pressure. Normal PA pressures are 15 mmHg to 30 mmHg systolic, 6 mmHg to 15 mmHg diastolic, and 9 mmHg to 17 mmHg mean. The normal oxygen saturation range is 70% ± 5%.

Abnormalities in the PA waveform and pressure readings can be caused by the following:

- Low pressure is seen in hypovolemia.
- Elevated pressure is seen in volume overload, pulmonary hypertension, and left heart failure.

About the Pulmonary Capillary Wedge Waveform and Pressure

The catheter is advanced with the balloon inflated into the pulmonary capillary wedge (PCW) position. A distinct change will be seen in the appearance of the waveform when it is in the PCW position. The waveform is similar in appearance to the RA waveform with distinct A and V waves and X and Y descents. The V wave is larger than the A wave.

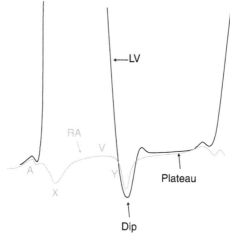

Figure 7.2 Simultaneous RA and LV pressure recordings demonstrating a dip–plateau pattern on the LV tracing, deep X and Y descents on the RA tracing, and equalization of diastolic pressures of the LV and RA. In early diastole, upon ventricular relaxation, there is a sharp decrease of ventricular pressure with subsequent sucking from the atria. However, the pressure in the ventricles quickly rises and equalizes with the pericardial pressure. This explains the *dip–plateau* (*square root*) shape of the RV and LV tracings in diastole and the *deep and rapid Y descent* on the RA and LA tracings during the early diastolic sucking. Y descent and the ventricular dip are superimposed. On the RA pressure, the A and V waves have equal height, corresponding to the pressure of the surrounding shell; this, along with the deep X and Y descents, gives the RA pressure tracing an M or W shape.

LA, left atrium; LV, left ventricle; RA, right atrium; RV, right ventricle.

Source: From Hanna, E. B., & Glancy, D. L. (2013). *Practical cardiovascular hemodynamics with self-assessment problems.* New York, NY: Demos Medical Publishing, LLC.

Normally, the pulmonary capillary wedge pressure (PCWP) is equal to or slightly lower than the PA diastolic pressure. PCWP reflects left atrial pressure (when the mitral valve is normal). Normal PCWP is 4 mmHg to 12 mmHg and it is recorded as a mean pressure. The normal oxygen saturation range for the PCW is 95% to 100%.

- A wave: It represents atrial contraction. The peak of the A wave occurs late in diastole and is aligned with the QRS complex on the ECG. It is not present in atrial fibrillation.
- X descent: It is the downstroke following the A wave and it represents the fall in pressure after contraction.
- V wave: It represents passive filling of the LA during systole. Its peak correlates with the opening of the mitral valve.
- Y descent: It follows the V wave and represents passive LA emptying.

Abnormalities in the PCW waveform and pressure readings can be caused by the following:

- Low pressure is seen in hypovolemia.
- Elevated pressure is seen in volume overload, left ventricle (LV) failure, mitral valve disease, cardiac tamponade, and restrictive cardiomyopathy.

Essential Facts

Right Heart Pressure Measurements
Normally the mean PCW = mean LA = left ventricular end-diastolic pressure (LVEDP).

These pressures may not correlate as closely in patients with mitral stenosis, severe mitral regurgitation (MR), aortic insufficiency, left atrial myxoma, severe LV noncompliance, and positive pressure ventilation.

A large V wave (greater than 10 mmHg) may be seen in acute decompensated MR because of the abrupt increase in the volume of the regurgitant flow into the LA. See Figure 7.3 to see an overall view of the hemodynamic tracings from the RA, RV, PA, and PCW positions. Figure 7.4 demonstrates the large V waves of mitral regurgitation.

LEFT HEART WAVEFORMS, PRESSURES, AND CALCULATIONS

About the Aortic Waveform and Pressure

To obtain aortic pressure, a catheter is advanced through the arterial sheath and placed in the aorta. The aortic waveform is composed of a rapid upstroke, indicating the beginning of systole, followed by a downslope. The dicrotic notch can be seen on the downslope and indicates closure of the aortic valve and the beginning of diastole. The aortic waveform is similar in shape to the PA waveform.

Aortic pressure is measured as a phasic (systolic, diastolic) and mean pressure. Normal systolic values are 90 mmHg to 140 mmHg, while normal diastolic values are 70 mmHg to 90 mmHg.

About the Left Atrial Waveform and Pressure

The left atrial waveform (see Figure 7.5) is similar to the RA waveform in that it consists of A and V waves and X and Y descents. It is typically slightly higher than the RA pressure. The LA is not routinely

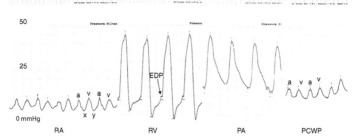

Figure 7.3 Right atrial, RV, PA, and PCWP tracings obtained while advancing the catheter from the RA to PA (50 mmHg scale). Mean RA pressure is equal to RV diastolic pressure, and mean PCWP is equal to PA diastolic pressure. Right atrial pressure and RVEDP are lower than PCWP and PA diastolic pressure, except in cases of "equalization of diastolic pressure" (tamponade, constriction, and severe RV failure).

Concerning RA and PCWP pressures: Note the A, X, V, and Y waves and the timing of the A and V waves (V peaks after T wave on ECG). *Concerning RV:* Note the rapidly upsloping RV diastolic pressure, particularly after the ventricular A wave, with a mildly increased RVEDP (10 mmHg), indicative of impaired RV diastolic function. The RVEDP corresponds to the peak of the electrocardiographic R wave and is the RV pressure seen after the A bump. *Concerning PA:* In contrast to the RV pressure that increases throughout diastole (upsloping) and has an A wave bump, PA pressure decreases throughout diastole (downsloping), does not have an A bump, and has a dicrotic notch. In contrast to the RA or PCWP tracing, the systolic PA peak occurs during ST/T interval, and the PA pressure is downsloping in diastole.

EDP, end-diastolic pressure; PA, pulmonary artery; PCWP, pulmonary capillary wedge pressure; RA, right atrium; RV, right ventricle; RVEDP, right ventricular end-diastolic pressure.

Source: From Hanna, E. B., & Glancy, D. L. (2013). *Practical cardiovascular hemodynamics with self-assessment problems.* New York, NY: Demos Medical Publishing, LLC.

accessed as part of a left heart cath procedure. Normal LA pressure is 6 mmHg to 12 mmHg. Normal oxygen saturation is 95% to 100%.

Access to the LA may be obtained during certain procedures, such as mitral valve valvuloplasty and repair, left atrial appendage occlusion, septal defect closure, and pulmonary vein (PV) isolation. To complete these procedures, a transseptal puncture and crossing of the septum is needed. Transseptal approach is further described in Chapter 8.

About the LV Waveform and Pressure

From the aortic position, the catheter is advanced over the aortic arch and through the aortic valve. In the absence of aortic stenosis (AS), the pigtail catheter generally crosses the aortic valve readily. The

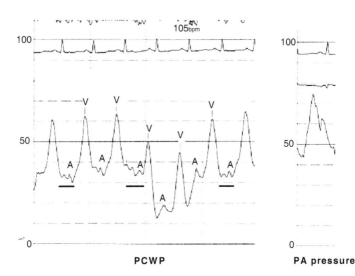

PCWP **PA pressure**

Figure 7.4 Another large V wave in a patient with severe MR. V wave amplitude is approximately 58 mmHg, whereas mean PCWP is approximately 38 mmHg (V wave > mean PCWP + 10 mmHg). To ensure it is V wave, note that it peaks after the end of the T wave on the ECG, there is a horizontal line between the waves (*black line*), A waves are seen, and the upstroke is more gradual than the downstroke, which is opposite to the PA tracing, wherein the upstroke is sharper than the downstroke.

MR, mitral regurgitation; PA, pulmonary artery; PCWP, pulmonary capillary wedge pressure.

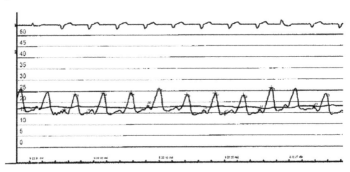

Figure 7.5 Left atrial pressure waveform with an elevated V wave due to mitral regurgitation.

waveform changes in appearance; a sharp upstroke is seen as the LV contracts and pressure peaks. The pressure then drops and diastole begins. In the LV, normal systolic values are 90 mmHg to 140 mmHg while normal end-diastolic values are 5 mmHg to 12 mmHg. Normal oxygen saturation is 95% to 100%.

LV systolic pressure is equal to the aortic systolic pressure, unless the patient has AS or a gradient within the LV itself. In AS, the valve is markedly narrowed, altering flow and causing a gradient or pressure difference between the aortic pressure and the LV pressure. With an intraventricular pressure gradient, pressures can be different within various areas of the LV, which can be seen in hypertrophic cardiomyopathy.

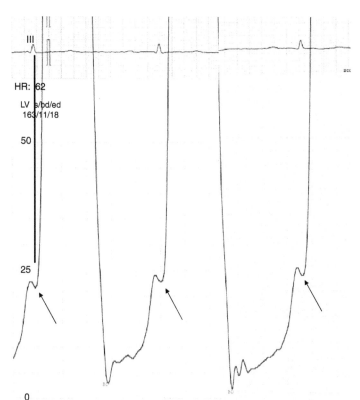

Figure 7.6 Normal mean LV diastolic pressure and normal LV diastolic pressure before the A wave. The LV pressure steeply increases during and after the A wave, leading to a pronounced A wave and a high LVEDP (*arrows*). This corresponds to the pattern of reduced LV compliance with compensated HF: Pre-A LV diastolic pressure and LA pressure are normal, but LV pressure sharply increases after atrial contraction.

How to measure LVEDP? (1) LVEDP coincides with the peak of the R wave on the ECG (*black line*); (2) LVEDP is the point on LV pressure tracing that follows the A "bump" (look for a bump on the LV upslope).

HF, heart failure; HR, heart rate; LA, left atrium; LV, left ventricle; LVEDP, left ventricular end-diastolic pressure.

Source: From Hanna, E. B., & Glancy, D. L. (2013). *Practical cardiovascular hemodynamics with self-assessment problems.* New York, NY: Demos Medical Publishing, LLC.

An important value that is obtained while the pigtail is in the LV is the end-diastolic pressure (LVEDP). It is measured just before the upstroke of systole, immediately after the A wave, if one is present (Figure 7.6). The LVEDP indicates LV preload and the health of the LV. It is elevated in volume overload, valvular stenosis, cardiomyopathy, and diastolic dysfunction. An example of a markedly elevated LVEDP is shown in Figure 7.7.

Table 7.1 summarizes the normal systolic, diastolic, and mean pressure readings in each heart chamber. It also indicates the normal oxygen saturation level that would be obtained if sampled.

Essential Facts

Know your patient's LVEDP—a normal finding is between 4 mmHg and 12 mmHg. It is an indicator of the overall health of the LV. If it is low, your patient may be hypovolemic and need fluids. If high, your patient may have heart failure and need a diuretic or vasodilator.

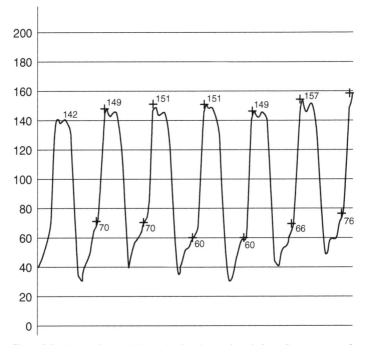

Figure 7.7 LV waveform with markedly elevated end-diastolic pressure of about 65 mmHg.

LV, left ventricle.

Table 7.1

Normal Heart Pressures and Oximetry

RA	RV	PA	PCW Lungs	AO	LA	LV
Mean pressure: 1–8 mmHg	Systolic pressure: 15–30 mmHg	Systolic pressure: 15–30 mmHg	Mean pressure: 2–10 mmHg	Systolic pressure: 100–140 mmHg	Mean Pressure: 2–10 mmHg	Systolic pressure: 100–140 mmHg
	Diastolic pressure: 1–8 mmHg	Diastolic pressure: 4–12 mmHg		Diastolic pressure: 60–80 mmHg		Diastolic pressure: 4–12 mmHg
70 ± 5%	70 ± 5%	70 ± 5%	95 ± 5%	95 ± 5%	95 ± 5%	95 ± 5%

Ao, aorta; LA, left atrium; LV, left ventricle; PA, pulmonary artery; PCW, pulmonary capillary wedge; RA, right atrium; RV, right ventricle.

Source: From Hanna, E. B., & Glancy, D. L. (2013). *Practical cardiovascular hemodynamics with self-assessment problems.* New York, NY: Demos Medical Publishing, LLC; Kern, M. J., Sorajja, P., & Lim, M. (2016). *The cardiac catheterization handbook* (6th ed.). Philadelphia, PA: Elsevier Saunders.

Chapter 7   **Cath Lab Hemodynamics: Waveforms, Pressures, and Calculations to Know**

ABOUT CO AND CARDIAC INDEX

CO is the volume of blood in L/min that is delivered to the body by the heart. The normal range for CO in the adult is 4 L/min to 8 L/min. It is calculated as heart rate multiplied by stroke volume. Stroke volume (SV) is the amount of blood ejected by the heart with each beat. Normal SV, depending on body size, is 60 to 130 mL. Determinants of SV include three things: preload, afterload, and contractility.

For example, if a patient's heart rate is 80 and the stroke volume is 70 mL, the CO is 5,600 mL/min or 5.6 L/min. When CO is corrected for body size, it is referred to as cardiac index (CI). The calculation for this is CO divided by the patient's body surface area (BSA). Normal CI in the adult is greater than 2.4 L/min/m^2.

- Preload: It is the volume of the blood coming to the heart to be ejected, or the amount of stretch on the myocardial muscle fibers at end-diastole. According to Starling's law of the heart, increased muscle stretch, up to a physiologic limit, results in a more forceful contraction and greater stroke volume for the subsequent beat. Preload can be manipulated. If a patient has low preload because they are hypovolemic, then the hypovolemia can be corrected by volume replacement with crystalloids, colloids, and/or blood. If a patient has high preload because the patient is volume overloaded, then that can be corrected pharmacologically using diuretics and/or vasodilating drugs.
- Afterload: It is the resistance to ejection, or the ventricular force or pressure required to overcome impedance to ejection. Afterload can be manipulated. If a patient has a low afterload because of sepsis, initial treatment is aimed at increasing the systemic vascular resistance (SVR), increasing preload, and administering inotropic agents. The underlying cause of the low afterload must be corrected. If the patient has high afterload, then the goal of therapy is to reduce the SVR. Nitroprusside, angiotensin-converting enzyme (ACE) inhibitors, and intra-aortic balloon pumping decrease afterload.
- Contractility: It refers to the pumping effectiveness of the LV. Contractility can be manipulated. If a patient shows signs of decreased contractility, the patient may benefit from inotropic agents. Inotropic therapy increases the strength of the contraction, increasing ejection fraction, stroke volume, CO, and tissue oxygenation.

Two commonly used techniques for measuring CO in the cath lab include:

- Thermodilution CO
- Fick CO

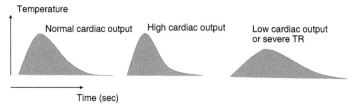

Figure 7.8 Temperature change at the tip of the PA catheter after injection of 10 mL of cold injectate. In case of high output, the cold injectate passes fast through the PA and is eliminated quickly. In case of low output, the temperature changes slowly, and a prolonged period is required for it to go up and then down, leading to a large area under the curve.

PA, pulmonary artery; TR, tricuspid regurgitation.

Thermodilution CO

The most widely used method to determine CO in the cath lab is the thermodilution method using a PA catheter. The PA catheter contains a thermistor located close to the distal tip of the catheter that assesses changes in temperature. When 5 mL to 10 mL of saline at a known temperature (usually room temperature) is rapidly injected into the proximal port, the thermistor detects this temperature change that occurs with the mixing of the saline and blood. The computer calculates this temperature change curve, plots a graph, and determines the area under the curve to calculate the CO. It is common that three injections with results within 10% of each other are averaged. Typical thermodilution CO curves are shown in Figure 7.8.

Thermodilution CO is most accurate in patients with normal or high CO. It may be inaccurate in patients with low-CO states (>3 L/min), shunts due to atrial or ventricular septal defects, severe tricuspid regurgitation, or an irregular rhythm.

Fick CO

The gold standard for measuring CO is the Fick principle in which CO is O_2 consumption divided by the difference between arterial and venous O_2. It was first described in 1870. Fick CO is useful for patients with:

- Shunts
- Low CO states
- Severe tricuspid regurgitation
- Irregular rhythm

To measure true Fick CO, the patient's oxygen consumption is measured using an oxygen analyzer placed around the head. Many cath labs are unable to perform true Fick CO easily so assumed Fick CO is calculated instead. The assumed value for oxygen consumption is typically 125 mL/min/m² or 110 mL/min/m² for elderly patients. The age cut-off for use of the "elderly" value is not defined in the literature.

To calculate an estimated Fick CO, the following is needed:

- Current hemoglobin
- Mixed venous (MV) blood sample from the PA
- Arterial blood sample

Cath Calculations: Assumed Fick CO Formula

$$\frac{O_2 \text{ consumption} \times BSA}{(A-V)O_2 \text{ difference} = (LV \text{ or aortic sat} - PA \text{ sat}) \times \text{Hemoglobin} \times 13.6}$$

Practice Data

BSA:	2.0 m²
Hemoglobin:	15 gm/dL
PA saturation:	60%
Aortic saturation:	99%
O_2 consumption:	125 mL/min/m²

$$\frac{(125 \text{ mL/min/m}^2) \times 2.0 \text{ m}^2}{(0.99 - 0.60) \times 15 \times 13.6} = \frac{250}{79.56}$$

Assumed Fick CO = 3.14 L/min

OXIMETRY RUN

Blood samples from various areas of the heart are obtained to localize the shunting of blood. A small sample of blood is drawn from the end-hole catheter and the oxygen saturation of the sample is measured. If there is an increase or "step-up" from the RA to the PA of greater than or equal to 7%, left to right shunting of blood may be present. When this step-up is present, a full saturation run should be done for a complete assessment of the abnormal shunting of blood. See Table 7.2 to understand where oximetry samples may be obtained. To be most accurate in measuring a shunt, all blood samples should be drawn within as short a period of time as possible.

Table 7.2

Full Oximetry Run for Shunt Assessment	
Low SVC	RV outflow tract
High SVC (near junction of RA)	Mid RV
High IVC	RV apex
Low IVC	Left and/or right PA
High RA	Main PA
Mid RA	Aorta
Low RA	

IV, inferior vena cava; PA, pulmonary artery; RA, right atrium; RV, right ventricle; SVC, superior vena cava.

Source: From Moscucci, M. (2013) *Grossman and Baim's cardiac catheterization, angiography, and intervention* (8th ed.). Philadelphia, PA: Lippincott, Williams, and Wilkins; Kern, M. J., Sorajia, P., & Lim, M. (2016). *The cardiac catheterization handbook* (6th ed.). Philadelphia, PA: Elsevier Saunders.

SHUNTS

Normally, pulmonary blood flow equals systemic blood flow. Pulmonary flow is represented as Qp while systemic flow is represented as Qs, so that Qp = Qs, normally a 1:1 ratio. When a shunt is present and there is abnormal flow, the normal 1:1 shunt flow ratio is disrupted.

Shunting occurs in:

- Atrial septal defects
- Patent foramen ovale
- Ventricular septal defects
- Patent ductus arteriosus
- Anomalous pulmonary venous return
- Tetralogy of Fallot
- Pulmonary atresia
- Transposition of the great vessels
- Truncus arteriosus

Shunts can be left to right, right to left, or bidirectional:

- In a left-to-right shunt, oxygenated blood shunts from the left heart or aorta to the right heart and mixes with venous flow. The shunted blood causes increased flow through the lungs so the Qp:Qs ratio is greater than 1:1. Qp:Qs greater than 1.0 indicates that a left-to-right shunt is present.

- In a right-to-left shunt, deoxygenated blood will shunt from the right heart or PA and mixes with arterial flow from the left heart or aorta. The shunted deoxygenated blood bypasses the lungs and enters the systemic blood flow, causing cyanosis. Qp:Qs less than 1.0 indicates a right-to-left shunt is present.

Cath Calculation: Shunt Calculation

$$\text{Formula for Qp:Qs} = \frac{(\text{Aortic saturation} - \text{MV saturation})}{(\text{PV saturation} - \text{PA saturation})}$$

- If the PV is not accessed, enter an assumed value of 98%.
- To determine the MV saturation, use the Flamm formula developed by Dr. Daniel Flamm, a Sacramento cardiologist who retired from the author's current facility.

$$\text{MV saturation} = \frac{3(\text{SVC sat}) + 1(\text{IVC sat})}{4}$$

Example:

SVC sat = 73%

IVC sat = 78%

$$\frac{3(73) + 1(78)}{4} = 74.3 = \text{MV saturation}$$

where MV = mixed venous, SVC = superior vena cava, and IVC = inferior vena cava.

CALCULATING THE AORTIC VALVE AREA

The Gorlin formula, first described in 1951, remains the standard formula for calculating the aortic valve area (AVA) in AS. The normal AVA is 3.0 cm^2 to 4.0 cm^2. Patients may not experience symptoms until the AVA is less than 2.0 cm^2. AS is considered critical when the AVA is less than 0.80 cm^2.

Factors that impact the AVA include the size of the opening, the flow across the valve, and the pressure gradient required to deliver that flow.

Information required to calculate the AVA includes:

- CO
- Gradient, or pressure difference, between the aorta and the LV
- Heart rate
- Time, measured as systolic ejection period (SEP)
- Gorlin constant for the aortic valve: 44.3

Two gradients are commonly determined during cath procedures: the peak to peak and the mean (Figure 7.9). The peak-to-peak gradient is the difference between the peak LV pressure and the peak aortic pressure. The mean gradient is the difference in pressure during the entire SEP and it is mathematically calculated by the computer. Using the calculated mean gradient is most accurate.

The gradient between the aorta and the LV can be measured in different ways:

- To obtain a pullback tracing, the physician will pull the catheter from the LV, back across the aortic valve, into the aorta while pressures are being recorded.
- Using a dual lumen pigtail, one port measures aortic pressure and the second port measures LV pressure.
- Using two transducers, obtain simultaneous pressure from a catheter in the aorta and a second catheter in the LV.

The SEP reflects the amount of time the aortic valve is open during each cardiac cycle. It begins when the aortic valve opens, indicated by when LV pressure exceeds aortic pressure, and ends when the aortic valve is closed or when aortic pressure exceeds LV pressure.

One version of the Gorlin formula for calculating the AVA is:

$$\frac{CO \ (in \ mL) \times Heart \ rate}{Square \ root \ of \ the \ mean \ gradient \times SEP \times 44.3}$$

When using the Hakki formula to calculate an approximate AVA, the formula is:

$$\frac{CO \ in \ L/min}{Square \ root \ of \ the \ peak\text{-}to\text{-}peak \ gradient}$$

Low Gradient AS

Dobutamine stress testing may be done to assess the efficacy of surgical or interventional aortic valve replacement for patients who present with a low aortic valve gradient and low CO. Coronary angiography

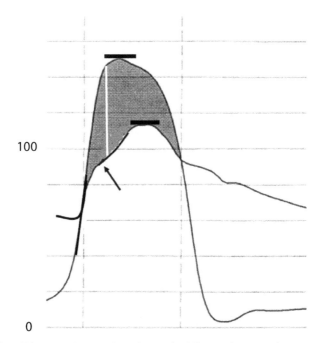

100

0

Figure 7.9 The peak-to-peak gradient is the difference between the two peaks (*black bars*), peak instantaneous gradient is the largest difference between the two *curves* (*white vertical line*), and mean gradient is the integration of all gradients under the *gray area*. LV pressure peaks early, and the aortic pressure peaks late, which is the opposite of what is found in HOCM. Note the anacrotic notch beyond which the aortic upstroke is slowed (*arrow*).

The mean gradient is usually close in value to the peak-to-peak gradient and is about 70% of the peak instantaneous gradient. The mean gradient is usually slightly smaller than the peak-to-peak gradient; however, in very severe AS with severely delayed aortic upstroke, the mean gradient area may end up being larger than the peak-to-peak gradient.

Note that in AS, the aortic pressure upstroke is less steep than the LV pressure upstroke; if the LV and aortic upstrokes are superimposed, suspect subaortic obstruction or error in zeroing creating a false gradient (i.e., the LV and aortic transducers were zeroed at two different levels).

AS, aortic stenosis; HOCM, hypertrophic obstructive cardiomyopathy; LV, left ventricle.

Source: From Hanna, E. B., & Glancy, D. L. (2013). *Practical cardiovascular hemodynamics with self-assessment problems.* New York, NY: Demos Medical Publishing, LLC.

should be done before the dobutamine infusion is started so that concomitant coronary artery disease can be determined. The presence of inotropic reserve, defined as an increase in stroke volume greater than 20% during dobutamine stimulation, is an important consideration when risk-stratifying a patient's operative risk.

CALCULATING MITRAL VALVE AREA

The Gorlin formula for the mitral valve is very similar to that of the aortic valve. The normal MVA area is 4.0 cm^2 to 6.0 cm^2. Patients may not experience symptoms until the MVA is less than 2 cm^2. Mitral stenosis is considered critical when the MVA is less than 1 cm^2.

Information required to calculate the MVA includes:

- CO
- Gradient between the LA and the LVEDP
- Heart rate
- Time, measured by the diastolic filling period (DFP) rather than SEP (Figure 7.10)
- Gorlin constant for the mitral valve: 33.7

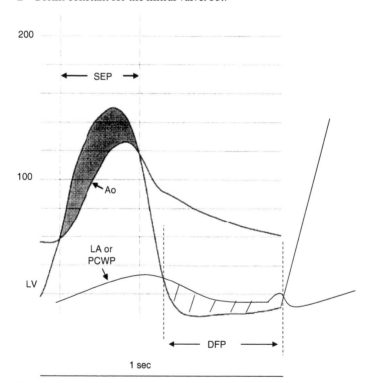

Figure 7.10 LV, Ao, and PCWP tracing in a patient with AS (LV–Ao gradient, *gray area*) and MS (PCWP–LV gradient in diastole, *dashed area*). Illustration of how to obtain SEP and DFP.

Ao, aortic; AS, aortic stenosis; DFP, diastolic filling period; LA, left atrium; LV, left ventricle; MS, mitral stenosis; PCWP, pulmonary capillary wedge pressure; SEP, systolic ejection period.

Source: From Hanna, E. B., & Glancy, D. L. (2013). *Practical cardiovascular hemodynamics with self-assessment problems.* New York, NY: Demos Medical Publishing, LLC.

Simultaneously recorded pressures of the LA/PCWP and the LVEDP are demonstrated in Figure 7.11. The shaded gray area indicates the gradient across the mitral valve due to mitral stenosis.

The DFP is the amount of time the mitral valve is open during each cardiac cycle. The gradient used in mitral valve calculation is the pressure difference between simultaneous LA and the PCW pressures, typically substituted by the PCWP and LVEDP. In the absence of mitral valve disease, the pulmonary wedge pressure (PWP) = LA = LVEDP.

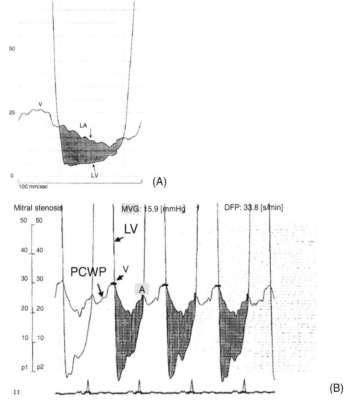

Figure 7.11 (A and B) Two cases of mitral stenosis with a diastolic pressure gradient between PCWP and LV at a heart rate of 70 bpm (*gray area*). Because of phase delay, the tracing of PCWP has been shifted to the left so that the peak of V, the wave is almost bisected by the LV downslope. There is no diastasis; LA pressure remains higher than LV pressure throughout diastole, signifying moderate or severe mitral stenosis. LA A wave is pronounced, but LV A wave is reduced because of ventricular underfilling.

DFP, diastolic filling period; LA, left atrium; LV, left ventricle; MVG, mitral valve gradient; PCWP, pulmonary capillary wedge pressure.

Cath Calculation: Gorlin MVA

$$\frac{CO \text{ (in mL)} \times \text{Heart rate}}{\text{Square root of the mean gradient} \times \text{DFP} \times 33.7}$$

SUMMARY

Hemodynamic assessment and calculations are an important part of many cath lab procedures. It is helpful to have a basic understanding of hemodynamics when you come into the cath lab setting. You will continue to grow and hone your knowledge of the interrelationship of pressure, flow, and resistance as you gain more experience and exposure to procedures.

8

Right and Left Heart Catheterization

One of the most basic and most common procedures performed in the cath lab is catheterization of the right and/or the left heart. Information and angiography images gleaned during these procedures are used in the diagnostic process to determine the best interventions. Understanding the indications and techniques for completing these procedures is essential.

In this chapter, you will learn:

1. Indications for right heart catheterization (RHC)
2. How an RHC is performed
3. Indications for left heart catheterization (LHC)
4. How an LHC is performed
5. When a transseptal approach is needed

RIGHT HEART CATHETERIZATION

In RHC a pulmonary artery (PA) catheter is advanced through a sheath in the femoral vein, right internal jugular vein, subclavian vein, or brachiocephalic vein and advanced to and through the right heart. Waveforms and pressures are recorded and measured as the catheter is advanced or as it is withdrawn. Blood samples may be drawn from various areas for oximetry. After pressures are recorded and cardiac output is measured, physiological data can then be calculated to assess the health of the right heart. RHC may not be done as a part of every diagnostic heart cath procedure. While the PA catheter can be placed at the patient's bedside without fluoroscopy, fluoroscopy is used to place it in the cath lab.

Indications

- Heart failure
- Cardiogenic shock
- Valvular heart disease
- Pulmonary hypertension

Contraindications

- Relative contraindications include active bleeding, severe anemia, severe electrolyte imbalance, sepsis, pregnancy, and recent stroke.
- Absolute contraindications include patient refusal and substandard imaging ability.

Complications

- Arrhythmias, including ventricular arrhythmias, heart block, and right bundle branch block (RBBB)
- PA rupture
- Pneumothorax (with internal jugular [IJ] or subclavian approach)
- Vascular complications at the access site
- Procedure-related complications are reviewed in detail in Chapter 12

Needed Equipment and Supplies

- A flow-directed PA catheter, commonly referred to as a Swan-Ganz catheter
- Fluid-filled tubings and transducers connected to the hemodynamic monitoring system
- Local anesthetic, needles, syringes, saline, sterile drapes

PA catheters are available in varying tip shapes, different numbers of lumens, and varying infusion ports (see Figure 8.1). Catheters are available with and without heparin bonding. A pacemaker option is also available. The distal inner lumen will accommodate up to a 0.025 inch (0.06 cm) guidewire, which may be needed to stiffen the catheter for better placement in some patients. If a guidewire is needed for a PA catheter, pull a J-tip rather than a straight guidewire to decrease the risk of wire perforation.

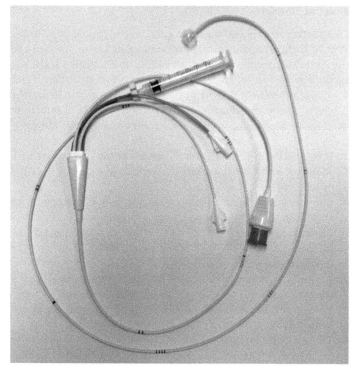

Figure 8.1 Pulmonary artery catheter.

Another available right heart catheter includes the Arrow–Berman catheter. It has side holes and is designed for pulmonary angiography. They are available in various Fr sizes and different lengths for use with pediatric and adult procedures.

Essential Facts

If your patient has a preexisting left bundle branch block (LBBB), monitor the patient very closely during the RHC. Why? The right bundle branch is located in the right ventricular (RV) endocardium and can be impacted by the passage of the right heart catheter. If the patient already has a LBBB, complete heart block or asystole can occur. Always ensure a temporary pacing wire, connecting cable, and temporary pacemaker generator are readily available in the procedure room.

Basic RHC Protocol

Choose the appropriate scale on your hemodynamic monitoring system. If right heart pressures are abnormally low or elevated and the entire waveform cannot be seen while on 50 mmHg scale, you should change to a different scale. Different scales available include 0 mmHg to 20 mmHg, 0 mmHg to 40 mmHg, 0 mmHg to 50 mmHg, 0 mmHg to 100 mmHg, 0 mmHg to 200 mmHg, or 0 mmHg to 400 mmHg, depending on your hemodynamic monitoring system.

1. Using sterile technique, flush all lumens of the PA catheter with saline prior to insertion. Test the balloon to ensure it does not leak.
2. The cardiologist manually advances the catheter antegrade, or with flow, through a venous sheath. Once the sheath is cleared, the balloon can be inflated and the catheter is advanced to the inferior vena cava (IVC). A blood sample for oximetry may be drawn from the IVC.
3. The catheter is then advanced into the right atrium (RA). The RA waveform is displayed and phasic and mean pressures (A wave, V wave) are recorded. A blood sample for oximetry may be drawn from the RA.
4. The catheter is then advanced through the tricuspid valve into the RV. The RV waveform will be seen on the monitor and phasic pressures (systolic, diastolic, and end-diastolic) are recorded.
5. The catheter is advanced until the waveform appearance changes into the pulmonary capillary wedge (PCW) waveform. The PCW waveform will be seen on the monitor and the A wave, V wave, and mean pressure are recorded. A blood sample for oximetry may be drawn from the PCW.
6. Deflate the balloon. The catheter is pulled back, through the pulmonic valve into the main PA. The PA waveform will be seen on the monitor and phasic and mean pressures are recorded. A blood sample for oximetry may be drawn from the PA.
7. Thermodilution cardiac output is done while the distal tip of the catheter is in the PA.
8. At the completion of the RHC, the catheter may be removed, or it may be left in place for continuing monitoring.

Please note that not all cardiologists do their RHC procedures in this specific order. Some may initially advance the PA catheter to the wedge position, measure the PCW, and then pull back the catheter chamber by chamber to obtain the remaining pressures.

LEFT HEART CATHETERIZATION

LHC is used to identify, evaluate, and treat:

- Coronary artery disease
- Valvular disorders
- Congenital heart anomalies

LHC is done by advancing a catheter retrograde, or against flow, through an arterial sheath, into the aorta, across the aortic valve, and into the left ventricle (LV). Waveforms and pressures in the aorta and the LV are recorded. Left atrial (LA) waveforms and pressures are not routinely measured unless the LA has been entered via a transseptal approach, described later in this chapter. The most commonly used catheter for this is a straight or angled (145°–155°) pigtail, which has an end-hole and multiple side holes.

Relative Contraindications

- Acute bleeding
- Recent intracranial hemorrhage
- Uncooperative patients

Complications

- Major complications are uncommon and include death, myocardial infarction, stroke, and serious arrhythmias requiring intervention.
- Bleeding, hematoma, and vascular injuries are the most common procedural complications.
- Procedure related complications are reviewed in detail in Chapter 12.

Needed Equipment and Supplies

- Needles
- Guidewires
- Sheaths
- Pigtail catheter
- Manifold system or power contrast delivery system
- Contrast, heparin

Essential Facts

When scrubbed in and assisting with procedures, do not advance a guidewire against resistance. Let the physician know that you are

(continued)

(*continued*)

meeting resistance. Resistance can indicate that there is an obstruction or that the guidewire is outside the inner lumen of the vessel. Advancing against resistance can also cause damage to the guidewire tip.

Basic LHC Protocol

The standard scale for LHC is 200 mmHg. The 20 mmHg or 50 mmHg scale is used when measuring the left ventricular end-diastolic pressure (LVEDP). If left heart pressures are abnormally elevated and the entire waveform cannot be seen while on 200 mmHg scale, change to a higher scale.

1. Obtain arterial access and place the sheath.
2. Heparin may be administered for anticoagulation.
3. Using sterile technique, flush the lumens of all of the catheters with saline prior to insertion.
4. The cardiologist manually advances the pigtail catheter over a guidewire through an arterial sheath. Never advance a guidewire against resistance. The guidewire is removed, and the catheter is flushed and attached to a pressure tubing connected to a transducer.
5. The aortic waveform is displayed. Phasic (systolic/diastolic) and mean pressures are recorded.
6. The pigtail is advanced through the aortic valve with the distal tip of the catheter located mid-cavity. Monitor closely for ventricular ectopy.
7. Measure/record LV pressures (systolic and end-diastolic) on 200 scale and 40 scale.
8. LV angiography may be done after pressures are recorded. The catheter is connected to a contrast line and the injection is done.
9. The pigtail catheter is removed and replaced with a coronary catheter (Figure 8.2). The coronary catheter is advanced over a guidewire.
10. The coronary artery is selectively engaged and angiography is performed via manifold or automated injector.
11. After all coronary views are obtained, record closing or ending aortic pressure (phasic and mean). Remove catheters.

Please note that not all cardiologists do their LHC procedures in this specific order. Some may wish to perform coronary angiography prior to measuring LV pressures and performing LV angiography.

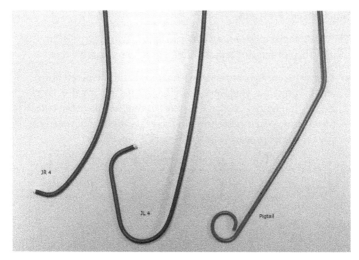

Figure 8.2 Commonly used catheters (left to right: JR 4, JL 4, pigtail).
JL 4, Judkins left 4; JR 4, Judkins right 4.

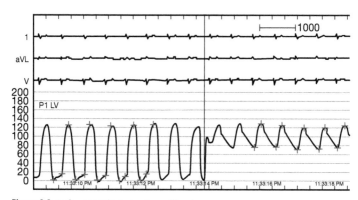

Figure 8.3 Left ventricle to aortic pullback.

LV Pullback

A quick way to assess for aortic stenosis (AS) is to look for differences in systolic pressure when pulling the pigtail catheter back through the aortic valve. In the normal aortic valve, there should be no gradient, or differences in systolic pressure. It is common to see artifact as the catheter is being pulled back, so this is generally not the best way to assess the aortic valve when AS is suspected (Figure 8.3).

Simultaneous Pressures

The cardiologist may request that you record two pressures simultaneously when evaluating a patient for a gradient across a value.

■ To most accurately evaluate for AS, record simultaneous aortic and LV pressures (Figure 8.4). In the normal aortic valve, there is little difference between the systolic components of the two waveforms. When AS is present, there is a gradient between the systolic aortic pressure and the systolic LV pressure.

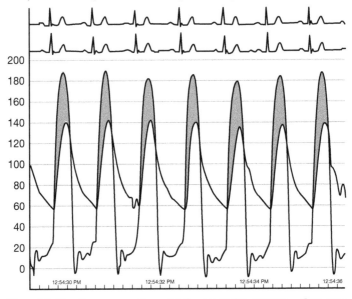

Figure 8.4 Simultaneous aortic and left ventricular pressures. Gray area represents the aortic valve gradient.

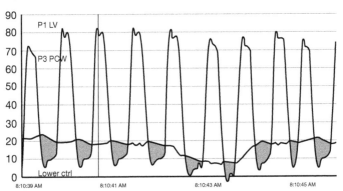

Figure 8.5 Simultaneous left ventricular and pulmonary capillary wedge pressures. Gray area represents the aortic valve gradient.

- To most accurately evaluate for mitral stenosis (MS), record simultaneous PCW and the LVEDP pressures (Figure 8.5). In the normal mitral valve, there is little to no difference between these two diastolic pressures. When MS is present, there is a gradient between the PCW and the LVEDP.

TRANSSEPTAL APPROACH

A transseptal approach is needed when access to the LA is needed. Procedures that require this include closures of an atrial septal defect or patent foramen ovale, mitral valvuloplasty, mitral valve clipping, occlusion of the LA appendage, and pulmonary vein isolation for arrhythmia ablation. Transseptal puncture is technically difficult and requires a skilled operator (Figure 8.6). The use of general anesthesia may be considered.

Contraindications to transseptal approach include:

- Uncooperative patients who cannot lie still
- Atrial thrombus
- Atrial myxoma
- Obstruction of the IVC

Commonly used equipment includes a transseptal Mullen's sheath and catheter or a Brockenbrough catheter, and transseptal needle.

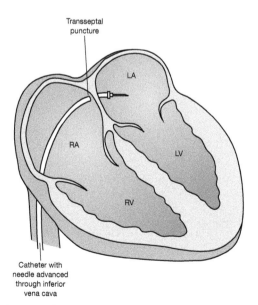

Figure 8.6 Transseptal approach.

The catheter and needle are placed via the right femoral vein, passing it into the RA and then crossing through the interatrial septum into the LA. Transesophageal echocardiography is commonly used for imaging of the catheter tip. An LA waveform will be seen as the needle and catheter cross the septum.

Heparin should be administered immediately to ensure clot does not form on the wires or catheters in the LA. LA pressure is measured and recorded.

Potential complications of the transseptal approach include:

- Puncture of the aortic root, coronary sinus, or atrial wall
- Cardiac tamponade
- Stroke, due to thrombus or air

SUMMARY

Learning to assist with a right and left heart cath is one of the basic steps when working in the cath lab. When you are scrubbing, you are at the table assisting the physician with catheter placement, performing cardiac output injections, drawing blood for arterial sampling, advancing and withdrawing guidewires, and injecting contrast. When you are in the monitoring role, you are recording the various waveforms and oximetry findings as well as entering the information required for various calculations done by the hemodynamic system. Your knowledge of normal and abnormal right and left heart findings is important to obtaining the optimal diagnostic findings for the patient.

9

Angiography

Angiography is commonly performed in the cath lab to visualize the coronary arteries, the various chambers of the heart, and the aorta. During your time working in the cath lab, you will see many angiographic images and initially it may be difficult to recognize what you are seeing. Listen to what the cardiologists and your team members are saying, ask questions when the timing is appropriate, review images as much as possible, and learn the tips and tricks outlined in this chapter.

In this chapter, you will learn:

1. Identifying normal coronary artery anatomy
2. Types of standard coronary catheters for femoral and radial approaches
3. Various x-ray views used in coronary angiography
4. Left ventricular angiography
5. Angiography of the aorta
6. How power injectors are used in the cath lab

ANATOMY REVIEW

The coronary arteries arise from the sinuses of Valsalva, located in the ascending aorta. They are located on the epicardial or outside surface of the heart and send perforating branches down into the myocardium. There are two major coronary arteries: the left coronary artery (LCA; Figure 9.1) and the right coronary artery (RCA; Figure 9.2).

Left Coronary Artery

- It arises from the left sinus of Valsalva.
- The initial segment of the LCA is named the left main (LM) coronary artery. The LM artery then bifurcates into the left anterior descending (LAD) and the left circumflex (LCx).
- The LAD follows along the anterior interventricular groove to the apex of the heart, supplying the anterior wall of the left ventricle (LV). It gives rise to the diagonal branches that supply blood to the lateral wall and the septal perforators that supply the septum.
- The LCx follows along the left atrioventricular groove, supplying the lateral wall of the LV. It gives rise to the obtuse marginals (OM). The initial OM branch is referred to as the first OM, the second as the second OM, and so forth.

Right Coronary Artery

- It arises from the right sinus of Valsalva.
- The RCA travels in the right atrioventricular groove and supplies the sinoatrial node in 60% of patients. The first branch of the RCA is the conus branch, which supplies the right ventricular outflow

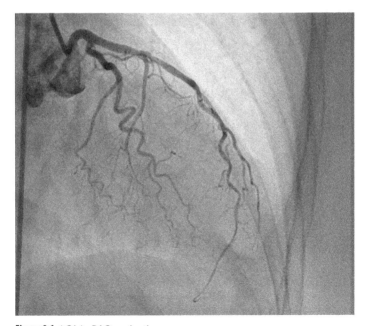

Figure 9.1 LCA in RAO projection.
LCA, left coronary artery; RAO, right anterior oblique.

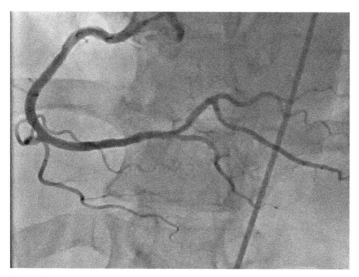

Figure 9.2 Right coronary artery in the LAO projection.

tract. The next branch of the RCA includes the sinus node artery, followed by the acute marginal branch and the atrioventricular nodal artery.

- Usually, the RCA bifurcates into the posterior descending artery (PDA) and the posterior lateral artery (PLA) in most of the population (85%). When this occurs, the patient is said to be "right dominant." In some patients (8%), the PDA and PLA come off the LCx, which would be referred to as a left dominant system. In a small number of patients (7%), the PLA comes off the LCx while the PDA comes off the RCA. This is called a codominant circulation.

Essential Facts

In about 20% of patients, there is an LM trifurcation rather than a bifurcation, and the vessel in between the LAD and the LCx is referred to as the ramus intermediate branch.

Coronary Dominance

Coronary dominance refers to the vessel that supplies the PDA. The majority of patients are right dominant, meaning that the RCA supplies the PDA. A small percentage (15%–20%) of the population is left dominant, with the LCx supplying the PDA.

DIAGNOSTIC CATHETERS FOR THE CORONARY ARTERIES

Diagnostic coronary catheters come in multiple sizes, pre-formed shapes and lengths, and are made by multiple manufacturers. Catheters are measured in French gauge sizes, most commonly abbreviated as Fr or F. French sizing was developed in the 1800s.

Essential Facts

French size is three times the diameter in millimeters; for example, a 6 Fr catheter is 2 mm in diameter.

Femoral Approach

For the femoral approach, 6 Fr diagnostic catheters are commonly used. Diagnostic catheters are also widely available in sizes 4 Fr through 8 Fr. The most commonly used coronary catheters are the Judkins left 4 (JL4) and Judkins right 4 (JR4). These catheters easily enter into or engage the coronary ostium in most situations. They are named after Dr. Melvin P. Judkins who developed them in the 1960s. The number following the *R* or the *L* indicates the curve of the catheter. A curve size of 4 works for most patients. For smaller aortic roots, 3.5 may be indicated; conversely if the aortic root is large, a 5 or 6 may be needed.

An alternative to the Judkins for a femoral approach is the Amplatz catheter, which is also available in multiple curve sizes. A left Amplatz 2 works for the LCA, a size 1 is needed for smaller aortic roots, and a 3 is needed for larger aortic roots. Right Amplatz catheters are also available for the RCA.

For saphenous vein grafts (SVG) from the femoral approach, the JR4, left coronary bypass (LCB), right coronary bypass (RCB), and internal mammary artery (IMA) catheters may be used.

Radial Approach

For radial approach, JL4 and JR4 coronary catheters may be used. There are also catheters available on the market that have been developed specifically for radial access. Examples of these include the Jacky, the Tiger, and the Sarah, and the Ultimate 1 and 2.

Essential Facts

Never advance a guidewire against resistance. If you meet resistance, stop and let the cardiologist know. Pass off the catheter/wire to the cardiologist to advance.

CORONARY ANGIOGRAPHY

Coronary catheters are advanced through the arterial access sheath over a 0.035 in. (0.09 cm) J-tipped guidewire and up into the aorta. Some cardiologists will want you to advance the guidewire around the aortic arch, while some will not. After the catheter is advanced, the guidewire is withdrawn. Wipe it with a wet sponge as it is removed. The catheter is then aspirated and flushed to remove any air. After flushing, the catheter is connected to the manifold/pressure injector system. An aortic waveform can then be seen and the pressure should be recorded.

Angiography of the coronary arteries is done to determine the origin, distribution, location, size, extent and severity of disease, and distal run-off or flow. During diagnostic cardiac cath procedures, multiple x-ray projections, angulations, or "views" of the coronary arteries are obtained to ensure that all segments of the artery are clearly seen without overlap.

The position of the x-ray source and the image detector to the patient is how projections are named, for example, left anterior oblique (LAO) or right anterior oblique (RAO).

Essential Facts

- LAO: The image detector is located on the patient's left side.
- RAO: The image detector is located on the patient's right side.
- Cranial: The image detector is tilted toward the feet.
- Caudal: The image detector is tilted toward the head.
- The angle of the image detector relative to the patient's midline further defines the view. For example, if the image detector is 30° to the left of the patient's midline, the view is described as 30° LAO.

Both the left and the RCAs are most easily cannulated in the LAO view. There are recommended standard views although individualization is needed. The first view of the LCA should look at the LM to assess for disease. The LCA is generally imaged in at least five views, including RAO caudal, RAO cranial, LAO caudal, LAO cranial, and lateral. The RCA is imaged in at least two views: LAO and RAO.

Essential Facts

Prior to an injection, the cardiologist may ask the patient to take a deep breath and hold it. This moves the diaphragm out of the view. Do not forget to remind the patient to breathe after the acquisition is completed!

Tips and Tricks for Identifying Coronary Arteries

- Look for the spine: The LCx will be closest to the spine in all views.
- In an LAO view, the spine will be seen on the right.
- In an LAO view, the apex of the heart points to the left.
- In an LAO view, the LAD is on the left and the LCx is on the right.
- In an RAO view, the spine will be seen on the left.
- In an RAO view, the apex of the heart points to the right.
- In an RAO view, the LAD is on the right and the LCx is on the left.
- In the AP cranial view and looking at the LAD, the septals go to the left and the diagonals go to the right.
- The RCA looks like the letter *C* in the RAO projection.
- The RCA looks like the letter *L* in the LAO projection.
- In cranial views, you should see the shadow of the diaphragm.

The catheter is advanced by the cardiologist into the aortic root and enters, or engages, into the coronary ostium, or opening. The catheter tip should be coaxial, or in the same plane, as the ostium. It is essential to look at the pressure waveform before injecting contrast. If damping or ventricularization of the pressure waveform is present, do not inject contrast. Injecting contrast when damping or ventricularization is noted can lead to coronary dissection, ischemia, or ventricular fibrillation.

Damping and Ventricularization

When a coronary catheter engages the ostium of the artery, the pressure waveform may become *damped* (Figure 9.3) or *ventricularized* (Figure 9.4) in appearance.

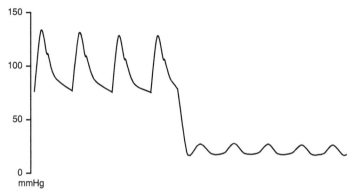

Figure 9.3 Damping of pressure tracing upon coronary engagement.
Source: From Hanna, E. B., & Glancy, D. L. (2013). *Practical cardiovascular hemodynamics with self-assessment problems.* New York, NY: Demos Medical Publishing, LLC.

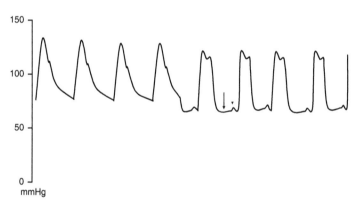

Figure 9.4 Example of ventricularization of the aortic pressure upon coronary engagement. The diastolic pressure does not necessarily drop to levels that are as low as the LA diastolic pressure, but the shape of the tracing changes from an arterial one to a ventricular one, that is, the diastolic segment between spikes is upsloping (*arrow*) and an A wave is seen (*arrowhead*).
LA, left atrium.

- In a damped pressure, there is a reduced systolic pressure at the catheter tip. It can indicate severe ostial disease or spasm, or the catheter is against the wall or a plaque.
- In a ventricularized pressure, there is a drop in the systolic pressure but a larger drop in the diastolic pressure. The waveform resembles a right ventricle (RV) or LV waveform. The catheter is likely obstructing antegrade flow. It typically indicates severe ostial occlusion.

Essential Facts

When injecting coronary arteries, perform the following:

■ Ensure the system is free of air.

■ Do not inject before the image acquisition begins.

■ Inject enough contrast to have some "reflux" of contrast into the aortic root.

■ If using a manifold, hold at a 45° angle so that any air goes away from the catheter.

■ For hand injections, build up the velocity of injection slowly and completely fill the artery, and ensure reflux of contrast around the ostium.

■ Too vigorous of an injection can cause coronary artery dissection.

■ Too long of an injection can cause bradycardia or ventricular fibrillation.

■ Watch the images while injecting, and then immediately look at the pressure after the injection is complete.

■ Spasm of a coronary artery can be induced by the catheter tip and this is seen most commonly with RCA cannulation. Coronary spasm is treated with nitroglycerin.

Coronary Collaterals

Collaterals are established channels that connect epicardial coronary arteries in response to myocardial ischemia (Figure 9.5). They can be ipsilateral—for example, the proximal RCA is filling the distal RCA—or contralateral, such as when a distal LAD is filling the RCA.

Anomalous Coronary Arteries

Anomalous, or abnormal, origins of the coronary arteries are uncommon (incidence <1.5%), but you will likely see some during your cath lab career. Many have no significant clinical impact.

■ The most common coronary anomaly is a separate origin of the LAD and of the LCx.

■ Another common anomaly includes the LCx arising from the RCA arising from the ascending aorta above the right sinus of Valsalva.

■ There are also significant anomalies that can lead to sudden cardiac arrest. These anomalies include the LCA arising from the right sinus and coursing between the pulmonary artery (PA) and

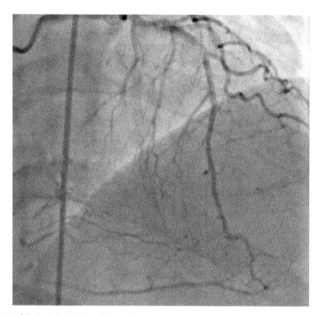

Figure 9.5 Left to right collaterals.

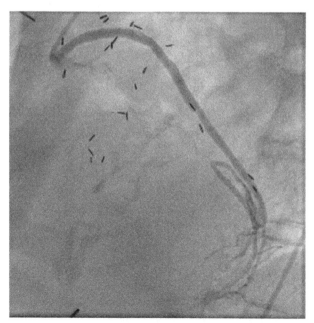

Figure 9.6 Saphenous vein graft.

the aorta (AO), the LCA arising from the PA, or a single coronary artery.

Myocardial Bridging

In myocardial bridging, portions of the normally epicardial coronary artery dip down into myocardium. It is a congenital coronary anomaly most frequently found in the LAD. The artery is then squeezed during systole and relaxes during diastole. Bridging can look like localized stenosis. Coronaries fill during diastole and most patients are asymptomatic. In severe cases, bridging can cause angina, arrhythmia, myocardial infarction, or sudden cardiac death because of direct compression of the artery.

ANGIOGRAPHY OF GRAFTS

Essential Facts

For patients who have undergone previous coronary artery bypass surgery, review previous angiograms whenever possible. If angiograms are not available, look for the surgeon's operative note to review the numbers of grafts and their location.

Saphenous Vein Grafts

Saphenous veins are commonly used as conduits in coronary artery bypass grafting (CABG). The vein grafts can develop disease, and at 10 years postplacement, only about 60% remain patent. Techniques for SVG angiography are similar to that of coronary angiography. RCA grafts can be best visualized in the LAO projection, while LCA grafts can be best visualized in the RAO projection. See Figure 9.6 for an example of an SVG angiography. While the most commonly used catheter is the JR4, other catheters used include the multipurpose (MP), modified right, and RCB or LCB catheters. Occluded grafts will usually appear as a stump (Figure 9.7).

Surgeons generally place the proximal anastomosis on the anterior surface of the ascending aorta, above the sinuses of Valsalva. While there can be variation, common placement is as follows: the highest on the aorta is usually the graft to LCx, the next lower one is usually to the diagonal branches, and then to the LAD, and the RCA is the lowest.

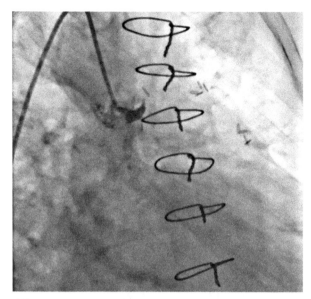

Figure 9.7 Occluded graft.

IMA Grafts

IMA grafts, especially the left IMA (LIMA), are commonly used as an arterial conduit in bypass surgery (Figure 9.8). They provide far superior long-term patency rates when compared to SVG. The LIMA arises from the left subclavian artery beyond the vertebral artery. An anteroposterior (AP) view is commonly used to cannulate. Catheters that may be used include the JR4 or an IMA catheter.

Radial Artery Grafts

Radial grafts are placed and cannulated similarly to SVG. They are smaller in diameter than SVGs.

Gastroepiploic Artery Grafts

The gastroepiploic artery is a branch of the gastroduodenal artery. Gastroepiploic artery grafts are rarely used now for bypass grafting. A Cobra catheter can be used to cannulate it.

ASSESSMENT OF CORONARY ARTERY STENOSIS

When cardiologists determine the degree of stenosis in a vessel, they are estimating it in relationship to the percentage reduction in the

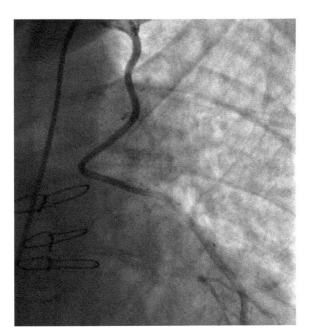

Figure 9.8 IMA graft.
IMA, internal mammary artery.

vessel diameter at its greatest narrowing. They are considering the extent and the severity of the narrowing. The LM is considered significantly narrowed when the lesion is 50% or more occluded. The LAD, LCx, and RCA are considered significantly narrowed when lesions are 70% or more.

The distal run-off of contrast is assessed and described based on standardized descriptors referred to as the *TIMI Coronary Grade Flow*, developed for an early thrombolysis in myocardial infarction clinical trial. See Table 9.1 for a more detailed description of TIMI flow.

Syntax Score

The Syntax Score is a complex validated tool developed to risk stratify patients according to the complexity and the extent of their coronary artery disease (CAD). It incorporates multiple factors, including:

- The number of lesions
- Lesion location
- Lesion length
- Presence of chronic total occlusion
- Bifurcations or trifurcations

Table 9.1

TIMI Coronary Grade Flow		
Grade	**Impact**	**Description**
TIMI 0	No perfusion	No contrast flow through the stenosis.
TIMI 1	Penetration with minimal perfusion	A small amount of contrast flows through the stenosis but fails to fully opacify the artery beyond.
TIMI 2	Partial reperfusion	Contrast flows through stenosis to opacify the terminal artery segment, but enters more slowly than the proximal segments. OR
		Contrast clears from a segment distal to stenosis more slowly than from a comparable segment not preceded by a significant stenosis.
TIMI 3	Complete reperfusion	Antegrade flow into the terminal artery segment is as prompt as antegrade flow into a comparable segment proximal to the stenosis. Contrast clears rapidly from distal segment as from an uninvolved, more proximal segment.

TIMI, thrombolysis in myocardial infarction.
Source: From Moscucci, M. (2013). *Grossman and Baim's cardiac catheterization, angiography, and intervention* (8th ed). Philadelphia, PA: Lippincott, Williams, and Wilkins; Topol, E. J., & Teirstein, P. S. (Ed.). (2016). *Textbook of interventional cardiology.* Philadelphia, PA: Elsevier.

- Aorto-ostial lesions
- Vessel tortuosity
- Calcification
- Thrombus
- Diffuse disease

An online algorithm is available at www.syntaxscore.com. The higher the score, the more complex the lesion(s). There is also a Syntax II score available, which adds in clinical information from the patient's presentation.

POWER CONTRAST INJECTORS

Power contrast injections are routinely used in the cath lab setting to rapidly inject large amounts of contrast for angiography to ensure optimal opacification. A power injector can deliver a larger amount of contrast over 2 to 3 seconds at a higher pressure. Coronary angiography can be completed using a manifold and hand injections, or it may be also be done using a power injector. The injectors may be freestanding or can be integrated into the table. Injectors are comprised of an injector head where the contrast is placed, a piston plunger that delivers the contrast, and pressure tubing that connects to the catheter. They are available from multiple manufacturers.

Injector parameters that can be adjusted include:

- Total volume and rate of contrast injected
- "Rate of rise" or the time in seconds until the peak injection rate occurs
- Pressure used for the injection, which is described in pounds per second (PSI)

When filling the injector, use care to ensure air is not introduced into the system. When connecting to the catheters, connect fluid-to-fluid to minimize the risk of air embolism.

LEFT VENTRICULOGRAPHY

Angiography of the LV is commonly performed during cath procedures. It provides valuable information regarding regional wall motion, ejection fraction (EF), and mitral valve function (Figure 9.9). A pigtail catheter is typically used for LV angiography. The pigtail catheter can be straight or angled (145° or 155°) with an end-hole and multiple side holes.

Good positioning of the pigtail catheter within the mid-LV is important. Ventricular ectopy can occur during positioning of the catheter but it does not typically require treatment other than repositioning the catheter. If the pigtail is too close to the mitral valve apparatus, it can cause artificial mitral regurgitation (MR) during the injection. If the pigtail is too close to the LV wall, excessive ectopy or LV staining can occur.

Common injector settings for LV angiography include:

- Rate of rise: 0 to 0.4 seconds
- Rate of injection: 10 mL/sec to 15 mL/sec
- Volume: 30 mL to 40 mL
- Maximum pressure: 1,000 PSI

Standard x-ray views for LV angiography include:

- 30° RAO: Best identifies the mitral valve and the high lateral, anterior, apical, and inferior walls of the LV
- 45° to 60° LAO with 20° of caudal angulation: Best identifies the aortic valve and the lateral, septal, and posterior walls of the LV

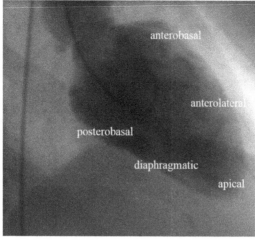

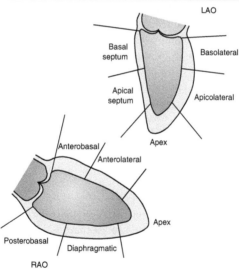

Figure 9.9 LV wall segments. Top image is LV angiography in RAO view. Bottom image shows ventricular wall segment names.

LA, left atrium; LAO, left anterior oblique; LV, left ventricle; RAO, right anterior oblique.

The competency of the mitral valve can be assessed during LV angiography. See Table 9.2 for standard grading descriptors. Normally, contrast should not be seen going from the LV into the LA during LV angiography. If the mitral valve is incompetent or regurgitant, contrast will be seen in the LA.

Cardiologists may choose to treat an elevated LV end-diastolic pressure with nitroglycerin prior to angiography. Nitrates reduce LV

Table 9.2

Quantification of Mitral Regurgitation

1+ MR: Faint opacification of the LA with clearing of contrast during each beat

2+ MR: Opacification of LA does not clear but is not as dense as LV

3+ MR: Opacification of LA is equal to that of the LV

4+ MR: Immediate dense opacification of the LA with filling of the pulmonary veins

LA, left atrium; LV, left ventricle; MR, mitral regurgitation.
Source: From Kern, M. J., Sorajia, P., & Lim, M. (2016). *The cardiac catheterization handbook* (6th ed.). Philadelphia, PA: Elsevier Saunders; Moscucci, M. (2013). *Grossman and Baim's cardiac catheterization, angiography, and intervention* (8th ed.). Philadelphia, PA: Lippincott, Williams, and Wilkins.

systolic pressure 10 mmHg to 15 mmHg and volumes by 30% to 35%. This unloads the LV and reduces the chance of contrast-induced pulmonary edema and volume overload.

Contraindications to LV angiography include patients who are hemodynamically unstable and patients with critical aortic stenosis, known LV thrombus, and/or a tilting disk prosthetic valve in the aortic position.

Complications of LV angiography include ventricular arrhythmias, heart block, endocardial staining, air embolism, and perforation with cardiac tamponade.

Essential Facts

Cardiologists may choose to omit an LV angiography for patients who have renal insufficiency to limit contrast intake. Echocardiography can be used to obtain information about LV function.

EVALUATING LV FUNCTION

Assessing the movement of the LV walls in systole and diastole provides information about wall motion and contractility. Descriptors used for describing LV wall motion abnormalities include:

- Hypokinesis: Wall motion is present but diminished.
- Akinesia: Wall motion is absent.
- Dyskinesia: Wall motion is paradoxical (abnormal outward movement during systole).

Unusual findings that can be seen with LV angiography include:

- Takotsubo cardiomyopathy
- Hypertrophic cardiomyopathy
- LV thrombus
- Ventricular septal defect
- LV aneurysm
- LV diverticulum

Ejection Fraction

EF is a measurement of global ventricular function and is calculated following LV angiography. EF is stroke volume (SV) expressed as a percentage of the end-diastolic volume (EDV). EF represents the ratio between the SV and the EDV. The EF is the percentage of the EDV that is ejected per beat. To obtain the most accurate EF, the systolic and diastolic contours of the LV are traced. The hemodynamic computer then calculates the EF. Many cardiologists can easily "eyeball" the angiography and estimate the EF.

Essential Facts

Normal EF is between 55% and 70%. An EF of less than 40% represents a clinically significant reduction in myocardial function.

Angiographic Cardiac Output

The angiographic cardiac output measures the total volume of blood ejected from the LV. SV can be determined by tracing the contours of end-diastole and end-systole. SV is the difference between the two. Once SV is calculated, that number can be multiplied by the heart rate to determine angiographic cardiac output. This method is rarely used as a primary way to determine cardiac output (CO).

AORTIC ANGIOGRAPHY

Angiography of the ascending aorta and the aortic arch may be done to evaluate:

- Aortic insufficiency (AI)
- Nonselective coronary or bypass graft visualization
- Aortic dissection or aortic aneurysm

- Aortic coarctation
- Atherosclerotic disease of the subclavian or carotid

For angiography of the ascending aorta and aortic arch, a pigtail is placed in the aorta with its distal tip just above the aortic valve. Using a pressure injector, 30 mL to 40 mL of contrast is injected over 2 seconds to 3 seconds at 1,000 PSI. An example of an aortic root injection can be see in Figure 9.10. Common x-ray views are 30° RAO for assessing AI and 40° to 60° LAO for identifying aortic dissection or visualizing the origin of vein grafts.

The aortic valve can also be easily assessed during angiography of the ascending aorta. In the patient with a normal aortic valve, no contrast should be seen in the LV during the injection of the ascending aorta. AI can be graded on a mild, moderate, severe scale or 1+ to 4+ scale. Refer to Table 9.3 for more detail.

Angiography of the abdominal aorta is done to evaluate:

- Renal and mesenteric vessels
- Abdominal aortic dissection or aneurysm
- Abdominal aortic and iliac atherosclerotic disease

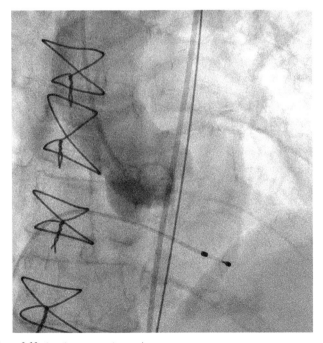

Figure 9.10 Aortic root angiography.

Table 9.3

Quantification of Aortic Insufficiency

1+ AI: A small amount of contrast appears in the LV during diastole, but clears with each beat

2+ AI: Faint opacification of the LV and contrast does not clear

3+ AI: Opacification of the LV is the same as opacification of Ao

4+ AI: Complete and dense opacification of the LV during diastole with the LV becoming more opacified than the Ao

AI, aortic insufficiency; Ao, aorta; LV, left ventricle.
Source: From Kern, M. J., Sorajia, P., & Lim, M. (2016). *The cardiac catheterization handbook* (6th ed.). Philadelphia, PA: Elsevier Saunders; Moscucci, M. (2013). *Grossman and Baim's cardiac catheterization, angiography, and intervention* (8th ed.). Philadelphia, PA: Lippincott, Williams, and Wilkins.

The distal tip of the pigtail catheter is positioned generally just above the renal arteries. A contrast volume of 25 mL to 40 mL is injected via a pressure injector over 2 seconds to 3 seconds. If digital subtraction angiography is available, less contrast can be used. Commonly used x-ray positions are anterior-posterior or a shallow LAO.

SUMMARY

After a short period of time in the cath lab, your comfort level with looking at angiography will improve. While it may take some time to identify the branches of the coronary arteries in the various views, with time it will become second nature. You will learn to identify areas of coronary artery stenosis, wall motion abnormalities, decreased EF, as well as normal and abnormal aortic and mitral valves.

10

Percutaneous Coronary Intervention

Percutaneous coronary intervention (PCI) is an umbrella term that includes several catheter-based techniques, including balloon angioplasty, stenting, atherectomy, and thrombectomy. PCI has become common treatment of coronary artery disease in the United States. First introduced in 1977, it has quickly evolved and become its own subspecialty in cardiology known as interventional cardiology.

In this chapter, you will learn:

- About the mechanism of balloon angioplasty
- Indications for PCI
- Medications commonly administered during PCI
- Equipment and supplies needed for interventional procedures
- Differences between bare metal stents (BMS) and drug-eluting stents (DES)

BALLOON ANGIOPLASTY

Percutaneous transluminal coronary angioplasty (PTCA) was the first catheter-based revascularization technique developed. Its development began in the 1970s by Dr. Andreas Gruntzig who performed the first in-man balloon angioplasty in 1977 in Zurich, Switzerland. In the early days of PTCA, the equipment was large and it was not unusual that mid-to-distal lesions could not be reached to be dilated.

Balloon angioplasty, now more commonly referred to as plain old balloon angioplasty (POBA), remained popular as primary treatment through the 1990s.

The limitations of POBA were its very high rate of restenosis (30%–50%) within the first 6 months of the procedure and severe dissections and perforations leading to abrupt closure in 5% to 10% of patients. Stents were originally developed to manage these mechanical complications of angioplasty. POBA by itself is rarely done anymore; stents are now placed in the majority of interventional procedures.

Interventional cardiology has developed its own language in regard to procedures, which can be confusing to a cath lab novice. Become familiar with the common key terms that you will hear. They are further described in Table 10.1.

Anatomy Review

The arterial wall is made up of three layers:

- Intima: The innermost layer, it is composed of squamous epithelial cells surrounded by connective tissue.
- Media: The middle and thickest layer, it is composed of smooth muscle.
- Adventitia: The outer layer, it is composed of connective tissue with elastic and collagen fibers.

Mechanism of Balloon Angioplasty

- Balloon inflation disrupts the plaque and arterial wall—causing fracturing and splitting, or dissection—of the intimal layer.
- Balloon inflation stretches the media, causing loss of elastic recoil.
- Balloon inflation pressure damages endothelial cells and compresses plaque.

CLINICAL INDICATIONS FOR PCI

- Angina not controlled by maximum medical therapy with evidence of ischemia such as an abnormal stress test
- Unstable angina, acute myocardial infarction (MI)
- Angina following bypass surgery
- Restenosis following previous PCI

Table 10.1

Key PCI Terms to Know	
Acute gain	The change in minimum lumen diameter from baseline to that immediately postprocedure.
ATM	Atmospheres of pressure.
Backing out	Guiding catheter is being pushed out of the ostium when pressure is applied to the balloon to advance it.
Back-up support	Ability of guiding catheter to remain seated properly and provide a stable base for movement of balloons and wires.
Balloon profile	Maximum diameter of the balloon before the balloon is unwrapped or expanded.
Balloon tip taper	Longer taper increases crossability of lesions.
Buddy wire technique	Done to help straighten the vessel if the stent will not advance on the guidewire. An additional guidewire (usually a heavier wire than the first) is advanced past the lesion and then the stent is advanced and the second wire is removed.
Coaxial alignment	Sharing the same axis; for example, the tip of the guiding catheter is in alignment or parallel to the ostium of the coronary artery.
Compliance	Ability of the balloon to increase in size with pressure.
Crossability	Ability to pass through the target lesion. Influenced by crossing profile and wrap profile.
Crossing profile	Largest portion of the distal catheter that must cross the lesion. Influenced by the marker bands and balloon bond.
Debulk	Removal of fibrous tissue, calcium, and thrombus on a lesion; often done prior to balloon angioplasty or placement of a stent.
Deep seating	Placing the guiding catheter past the ostium and into the vessel to obtain better support for crossing lesions. Increases risk of catheter-induced dissections.
Deliverability	Ability to reach the target lesion. Influenced by pushability and trackability.
Direct stenting	Stent deployment is done without predilation of the lesion.
Dog-boning	Expansion of an angioplasty balloon at the proximal and distal ends, likened to a dog bone shape. Results in suboptimal expansion of the stent. More common with compliant balloons.

(continued)

Table 10.1

Key PCI Terms to Know (continued)

Kissing balloons	The simultaneous inflation of two side-by-side angioplasty balloons, with one in the main branch of a bifurcation and the other in the side branch.
Late loss	Difference in minimal luminal diameter between procedure end and follow-up.
MACE	Acronym for major adverse cardiac events
Negative prep	Balloon is aspirated only; helps maintain a smaller profile.
Nominal pressure	Amount of pressure in ATM required to inflate the balloon to its labeled diameter.
Nominal size	Stated diameter and length a balloon should reach when dilated to nominal pressure.
Noncompliant	Balloon that increases less than 10% when inflated above its nominal pressure.
Plaque shift	Displacement of plaque during balloon inflation.
Positive prep	Balloon is aspirated, inflated with contrast, and then aspirated again to remove any air.
Profile	Maximum cross-sectional diameter of the balloon.
Pushability	Transmission of forward push force from proximal end to distal end. Influence by shaft column strength, kink resistance, and wire compatibility. OTW delivery systems provide greater pushability than RXx delivery systems.
Radial force	Force exerted on the lesion and vessel wall by the inflated balloon. Influenced by balloon compliance.
Rated burst pressure	The pressure level in ATM the balloon is designed to be inflated without rupturing.
Snow plow injury	Plaque shifting at the carina of a bifurcation where plaque is moved into the ostium of the side branch.
Torque	Turning, twisting.
Trackability	Ease with which the balloon catheter follows over the guidewire into the coronary arteries. Influenced by friction, catheter profile, and catheter flexibility.
Waist	Hourglass appearance with central restriction.
Watermelon seeding	Tendency of an inflated balloon to slip within the lesion.
Working length	Balloon surface in contact with intima when inflated.
Wrap	Tightness of balloon material wrapped around the shaft of the balloon catheter when manufactured.

OTW, over the wire, PCI, percutaneous coronary intervention.

MEDICATIONS COMMONLY USED IN PCI

Anticoagulation

Anticoagulation is indicated for most procedures to decrease the risk
of thrombus formation during procedures. Unfractionated heparin
and bivalirudin are most commonly used. Refer to Table 10.2 for
more information on anticoagulants. Bleeding is the most common
adverse effect of anticoagulation therapy.

During PCI, the administration of unfractionated heparin is
guided by the activated clotting time (ACT).

ACT is a point-of-care lab test done in the cath lab to assess the
effects of anticoagulant administration, especially heparin. It can be
done to measure anticoagulation from bivalirudin also, but it is less
accurate. ACT measures the amount of time it takes whole blood to

Table 10.2

Medications Used for Anticoagulation

	Typical Dosing	Nursing Implications
Unfractionated heparin	For interventional procedures: 70–100 units/kg if no concomitant IIb/IIIa GPI to achieve desirable ACT range.	Monitor ACT. Reduce to 50–60 units/kg when concomitant IIb/IIIa GPI given. No renal dose adjustment is needed. Can be reversed with protamine. Can cause heparin-induced thrombocytopenia.
Bivalirudin (Angiomax)	For interventional procedures: Initial bolus of 0.75 mg/kg followed by IV infusion of 1.75 mg/kg/hr for at least the duration of the PCI. Checking ACT 5–10 min after administration confirms its administration.	Direct thrombin inhibitor. Associated with significantly reduced risk of 30-day mortality after primary PCI. Risk of acute stent thrombosis is highest in 4 hours after primary PCI. Monitor aPTT and ACT. Renal dose adjustment is needed.
Enoxaparin (Lovenox)	Without IIb/IIIa GPI: 1 mg/kg IV. With IIb/IIIa GPI: 0.5–075 mg/kg IV.	Low molecular weight heparin. Renal dose adjustment is needed. Does not reliably impact ACT. Can be partially reversed with protamine.

ACT, activated clotting time; aPTT, activated partial thromboplastin time; GPI,
glycoprotein inhibitor; IV, intravenous; PCI, percutaneous coronary intervention.

clot when exposed to a substance like celite or kaolin. The longer the blood takes to clot, the higher the value. It is reported in seconds.

- Check ACT 5 to 10 minutes after heparin administration and then every 30 minutes or so.
- Target ACT for PCI is around 250 seconds. If target ACT is not met, additional heparin should be administered.

Antiplatelet Therapy

The treatment of coronary and peripheral artery disease with antiplatelet agents is required to prevent the activation and aggregation of platelets, which leads to thrombus formation. Aspirin is a potent antiplatelet drug and is usually a lifelong drug for patients following PCI and coronary bypass surgery. $P2Y^{12}$ inhibitors are routinely required following PCI and many patients are continued for 12 months. Table 10.3 outlines the commonly used antiplatelet agents. The concurrent dosing of aspirin and a $P2Y^{12}$ inhibitor is referred to as dual antiplatelet therapy (DAPT). Bleeding is the most common adverse reaction of antiplatelet therapy.

Table 10.3

Antiplatelet Agents		
	Typical Dosing	Nursing Implications
Aspirin	325 mg PO before PCI followed by 81–325 mg PO daily.	Rapidly absorbed; achieves peak plasma levels within 30 minutes. 5%–60% of patients may be nonresponders. If allergic, use clopidogrel; if time permits, perform ASA desensitization using escalating doses.
$P2Y^{12}$ Inhibitors		
Ticagrelor (Brilinta)	Loading dose 180 mg PO followed by 90 mg PO twice daily. Maintenance ASA dosing recommended is 81 mg/day.	More rapid onset of action than clopidogrel. Reversible. Can induce dyspnea, hyperuricemia, and ventricular pauses in some patients.
Clopidogrel (Plavix)	Loading dose 300–600 mg PO followed by 75 mg PO daily.	Some patients are nonresponders.
Prasugrel (Effient)	Loading dose 60 mg PO followed by 10 mg PO daily.	More rapid onset of action than clopidogrel.

(continued)

Table 10.3

Antiplatelet Agents (*continued*)	Typical Dosing	Nursing Implications
Cangrelor (Kengreal)	30 mcg/kg IV bolus followed by 4 mcg/kg/min continuous infusion.	Direct inhibitor of the P2Y^{12} platelet receptor. Platelet inhibition occurs within 2 minutes of administration. Infusion should be continued for 2 hours or the duration of the PCI, whichever is longer. After discontinuation, platelet function returns to normal within 1 hour. Transient dyspnea can occur in some patients.

ASA, acetylsalicylic acid; PCI, percutaneous coronary intervention; PO, per os.

Table 10.4

Glycoprotein IIb/IIIa Inhibitors	Typical Dosing	Nursing Implications
Abicximab (Reo-Pro)	0.25 mg/kg IV bolus followed by 0.125 mcg/kg/min (max: 10 mg/min) IV infusion for 12 hours.	Murine monoclonal antibody; allergic reaction possible. Functional half-life of up to 7 days. Can cause profound thrombocytopenia quickly. No renal dose adjustment is needed. Can be reversed with platelet administration.
Epitifibatide (Integrilin)	180 mcg/kg IV × 2 (max: 22.6 mg), 10 minutes apart and 2 mcg/kg/min infusion (max: 15 mg/hr) for minimum of 12 hours.	Renal dose adjustment is needed. Platelets recover within 4 hours of stopping infusion.
Tirofiban (Aggrastat)	25 mcg/kg bolus followed by 0.15 mcg/kg/min infusion for up to 18 hours.	Renal dose adjustment is needed. Ninety percent platelet inhibition within 10 minutes of administration. Platelets recover within 4–8 hours of stopping infusion.

Glycoprotein IIb/IIIa Inhibitors

Inhibitors of the IIb/IIIa glycoprotein block the final common pathway of platelet aggregation by binding fibrinogen. They are predominately used for the high-risk acute coronary syndrome (ACS) patient with elevated biomarkers. Refer to Table 10.4 for further details.

When using IIb/IIIa glycoprotein inhibitor (GPI) agents, an ACT of 200 seconds is sufficient. Dosing of heparin should be reduced when IIb/IIIa GPI are used. Bleeding is the most common adverse reaction of all IIb/IIIa GPI agents.

EQUIPMENT AND SUPPLIES NEEDED FOR PCI

- Sheaths: 6 to 7 Fr sizes commonly used
- Guiding catheters, also called guides: 6 to 7 Fr sizes commonly used
- Coronary guidewires: 0.014 inch (0.035 cm) commonly used
- Balloon catheters: Multiple sizes and lengths are available
- Stents: Multiple sizes and lengths are available
- Accessories including indeflators, rotating hemostatic valve or Tuohy–Borst valve, torque device, and guidewire introducer

More About Guiding Catheters

- Available in multiple pre-formed shapes, similar to coronary diagnostic catheters.
- Standard length is 100 cm.
- Provides stable support for advancing and delivering guidewires and balloons to and across the lesion.
- Has a softer atraumatic tip, larger inner lumen, and stiffer shaft than a diagnostic catheter.
- Constructed of an outer protective layer, the core is stainless steel or Kevlar to provide stiffness and torque and the inner coating is polytetrafluoroethylene (PTFE) or silicone to promote easy passage of wires and devices.
- Allows for pressure monitoring and contrast delivery around the balloon angioplasty catheter.
- May have side holes to allow for distal coronary flow.

More About Coronary Guidewires

- Available in various sizes, 0.010 inch to 0.018 inch (0.025 cm to 0.045 cm) with 0.014 inch (0.035 cm) most commonly used in PCI.
- Available in two different lengths: 140 to 175 cm and 280 to 300 cm (exchange).
- Required to cross the lesion atraumatically to provide access for balloons and stents.
- Many different guidewires are available; they vary in tip softness, trackability, steerability, torque control, flexibility, support, stiffness, and visibility during x-ray imaging.

- Core can be steel or nitinol.
- J tip can often be reshaped.
- May have radiopaque markers (gold or platinum) to improve visibility.
- May be coated with silicone, heparin, PTFE, or Teflon; hydrophobic (repels water) or hydrophilic (attracts water)
- Workhorse or frontline guidewires; most physicians have a preferred workhorse guidewire: softer tips and medium support for the bulk of the work. Examples include Balance Middle Weight (BMW), Prowater Flex, High Torque Floppy, Cougar, and Runthrough.
- Extra support guidewires have a stiffer shaft and are better for use in tortuous or calcified lesions.

More About Angioplasty Balloons

- Wide variety of sizes and balloon lengths available.
- May be over-the-wire (OTW) or rapid exchange (RX)/monorail design. Fixed-tip balloon catheters are rarely used now.
  - OTW system has dual lumen with ports for guidewire and balloon inflation. Length: 145 cm to 155 cm. A guidewire can be advanced from either end. They have a slightly large profile. They may have more pushability. Need two operators and there may be slightly more fluoroscopy time with their use.
  - RX balloons are designed for single-operator use, allowing quicker exchanges over a shorter wire. Exchanges are quicker, resulting in less fluoroscopy time. The catheter can have less pushability.
- Compliance is an important characteristic of angioplasty balloons.
  - Compliant balloons will predictably increase or overstretch up to 20% of stated nominal size with increased pressure.
  - Noncompliant balloons are stiffer and made to withstand high pressures and will not increase or overstretch with increasing pressure. They are useful for poststent dilation as well as calcific lesions, hard-to-dilate lesions, and aorto-ostial lesions.
- Balloon prep
  - Positive prep: Aspirate balloon, inflate with 50/50 contrast, and then aspirate again to remove any air.
  - Negative prep: Aspirate balloon with contrast-filled syringe, and then allow a small amount of contrast into the balloon when the syringe is released; negative prep maintains the lowest balloon profile.
  - Refer to the instructions for use (IFU) to review the manufacturer's recommendations.

More About Stents

- Come in multiple sizes, lengths, and thicknesses.
- Stents are made of metal, such as stainless steel, cobalt chromium, platinum, and nitinol or may have bioabsorbable scaffolding.
- Can be coated with a drug-eluting polymer.
- Available as balloon expanding or self-expanding.
  - Balloon-expanding stents are mostly commonly used for coronary stenting.
  - Self-expanding stents are mostly used for saphenous vein grafts and carotid, iliac, and femoral stenting.
- Stent strut design: Coil, slotted tube (closed cell and open cell), or modular.
  - Closed cell: Less space per cell, higher metal-to-artery ratio, improved scaffolding, greater radial strength.
  - Open cell: More space between struts, more flexible, greater flexibility.

More About Needed Miscellaneous Supplies

- Indeflator: Needed to inflate the balloon and provide precise measurement of balloon inflations in atmospheres of pressure (ATM).
- Hemostasis valve/Y connector: Connects to the hub of the guiding catheter and allows the entry of the balloon while minimizing back bleeding; allows pressure measurement and contrast injection.
- Torque tools: Attach to the wire and allow the operator to turn the wire.
- Diluted contrast: For balloon inflation, 50/50 dilution with saline is common.

PCI PROCEDURE STEPS

1. Arterial access is obtained.
2. Anticoagulation is administered to obtain target ACT greater than 200 seconds.
3. The guiding catheter, also referred to as a guide, is selected and prepared for entry through the arterial sheath. The catheter is advanced over the larger 0.35 inch (0.875 cm) guidewire. The catheter is positioned near the coronary ostium and the guidewire is removed.
4. The coronary artery is cannulated and initial angiography is recorded. These images, commonly referred to as guiding

shots, are used as a reference or road map for wire and balloon placement.

5. A 0.014 to 0.018 inch (0.035 to 0.045 cm) guidewire is introduced into the catheter and advanced into the coronary artery. The guidewire is advanced across the lesion.

6. An angioplasty balloon catheter is placed over the guidewire and advanced through the guiding catheter to the lesion.

7. When optimally positioned at the lesion, the balloon is inflated using the indeflator. The lesion is expanded by balloon inflations.

8. Leaving the guidewire in place with the tip of the wire distal to the lesion, the angioplasty balloon catheter is then removed.

9. An angioplasty balloon mounted with a stent is then advanced over the guidewire and positioned at the lesion.

10. The balloon is inflated, as previously mentioned, which expands and deploys the stent. High pressure should be used to expand the stent fully. The balloon is deflated and the catheter is removed, leaving the guidewire in place.

11. Angiography is completed to assess stent placement. If results are satisfactory, the guidewire is removed and final angiography is completed, and then the guiding catheter is removed.

Essential Facts

Keep the distal tip of the guidewire stationary during angioplasty and stent catheter exchanges.

- Develop a system for managing multiple guidewires and balloons on the table: Wipe with a wet four-by-four sponge, rehoop if possible, and keep the tip protected.
- Visually and verbally confirm balloon and stent sizes when passed by the circulator.
- When estimating vessel size, remember that a 6 Fr guide = 2 mm.

MORE ABOUT CORONARY STENTING

Stents were initially developed in the 1980s as a way to prevent abrupt closure from balloon-induced dissections by providing a scaffold to physically hold open the vessel. Early clinical trials found significant reductions in restenosis rates in the stent group compared to the POBA group. Although restenosis was reduced, stent usage led to the development of in-stent restenosis (ISR), which occurred in about

20% to 30% of patients. ISR is caused by neointimal hyperplasia due to proliferation and migration of vascular smooth muscle cells, leading to scar tissue within the stent. The use of stents remains limited by vessel size and anatomy. Vessels smaller than 2 mm are not suitable for stenting. Vessel segments that are tortuous, angulated, and/or calcified can be difficult to stent.

Optimal Stenting Technique

- Balloon predilation is commonly done prior to stent deployment. It helps with delivery and deployment of the stent. The delivery of a stent without predilation is called *direct stenting*. It can be successful in larger vessels and proximal lesions and if there is no calcification or angulations.
- The full expansion of all stent struts is essential for success. Stent underexpansion has been associated with ISR and abrupt stent thrombosis. The entire lesion and the area of barotrauma caused by the balloon inflation needs to be covered by the stent.
- Postdilation is often done with an appropriately sized high-pressure balloon at 12 ATM to 16 ATM of pressure to fully expand stent struts. Lower pressures, 8 ATM to 14 ATM, may be used when the vessel tapers.
- Suboptimal stenting leads to poorer patient outcomes, such as an increase in rate of non–ST-segment elevation myocardial infarction (STEMI), restenosis, and increased major adverse cardiac events (MACE).

Drug-Eluting Stents

Interest in developing a stent that would reduce ISR lead to the development of the DES. Stent polymer coatings are applied to stainless steel, cobalt-chromium, and nickel-chromium stents, allowing for the controlled release of a drug that decreases ISR. These polymers elute drug over weeks to months. Chemotherapy-type drugs are used, including sirolimus and paclitaxel. Newer drugs, zotaroliumus and everolimus, are analogs of sirolimus.

Essential Facts

Patients who receive DES need prolonged aspirin and an ADP receptor antagonist like ticagrelor or clopidogrel. This is referred to as (DAPT) and it should be continued for 12 months following DES placement.

Bare Metal Stents

While the majority of stents used in the United States today are drug eluting, there remains a place for the use of BMS for some patients. Indications for the use of BMS include:

- Active bleeding or very high risk of bleeding at the time of PCI
- Noncardiac surgery planned within 6 weeks of PCI
- History of medication noncompliance
- Very large vessel size (>5 mm) where the rate of restenosis with BMS is low

Bioabsorbable Stents

Bioabsorbable stents have been developed but have not been found to be superior to everolimus-eluting stents. They have been found to be associated with late and very late stent thrombosis. Continuing research and development is needed.

Covered Stents

Covered stents are used to close artery perforations and stop hemorrhage. Stainless steel balloon-expandable stents are covered with a PTFE membrane between them. They are available commercially as the Graftmaster RX coronary stent graft (Abbott).

OTHER INTERVENTIONAL MODALITIES

POBA and stenting may be performed in conjunction with other modalities such as atherectomy or thrombectomy to debulk lesions to remove calcium, fibrosis, or thrombus prior to stent placement.

Atherectomy

Techniques for atherectomy, or removal of plaque from the lesion, were developed in the 1980s as a way to modify plaque to decrease restenosis. Different techniques are available including directional, rotational, orbital, and laser atherectomy.

Directional Atherectomy

- The first atherectomy device was the Simpson AtheroCath, which received the Food and Drug Administration's approval in 1990. It worked by cutting away plaque and collecting the plaque into the nose cone of the catheter. The device would then be rotated to cut more plaque. This technique was referred to as directional coronary atherectomy (DCA). The AtheroCath is no longer available.

- The current DCA device is the SilverHawk catheter (Medtronic). It removes tissue through cutting and retrieval.

Rotational Atherectomy

- Available as the Rotablator (Boston Scientific), developed in 1988. It uses a nickel-plated brass burr encrusted with diamonds that rotates between 140,000 and 200,000 rounds per minute (RPM). It is powered by compressed nitrogen.
- Removes fibrocalcific plaque to debulk the vessel before stenting is done.
- Works on the principle of differential cutting; soft tissues are not injured by the rotating burr.
- Requires use of specific guidewires (RotaFloppy guidewires).
- Produces microparticles that can lead to slow flow or no flow.
- A mixture of vasodilators can be used as a flush to decrease the spasm and no-reflow phenomenon. Nitroglycerin, heparin, verapamil, and adenosine may be used for this. Rotoglide (Boston Scientific) may be added to decrease friction and heat buildup. Rotoglide should not be used if the patient is allergic to eggs or olive oil.
- Consider backup temporary pacemaker for right coronary artery (RCA) and dominant left circumflex (LCx) lesions. Aminophylline 200 mg to 300 mg may be used to prevent bradycardia.

Orbital Atherectomy

- Commercially available as the Diamondback 360° (Cardiovascular Systems, Inc.).
- Eccentrically mounted diamond-coated crown that rotates in an elliptical orbit over a guidewire; speeds ranging from 60,000 RPM to 200,000 RPM.
- Based on the principle of differential sanding and centrifugal force.
- Provides bidirectional cutting.
- Microparticles produced are smaller than those produced in rotational atherectomy.

Laser Atherectomy

- Laser light energy can be used to vaporize plaque, thrombus, and neointimal hyperplasia.
- The currently available system is the Excimer laser system (Specranetics).

- The laser beam is transmitted through the catheter and is pulsed in bursts at a controlled energy level and frequency. It is referred to as *fluence* and is measured in Hz.

Cutting/Scoring Balloons

- Specialty catheter with three to four small blades designed to make controlled incisions into lesions, also referred to as controlled dissection.
- Current products include the Wolverine Cutting Balloon (Boston Scientific) and the Angiosculpt scoring balloon (Spectranetics).
- Useful for tough fibrous intimal hyperplasia.
- Indicated for ISR, undilatable lesions, bifurcation lesions, and ostial lesions.
- Best for short concentric lesions when thrombus is not present.
- Best to slowly inflate and deflate to allow to unfold and rewrap properly.
- Inflate for 60 second to 90 seconds to ensure time for cutting, also referred to as scoring.

Thrombectomy

Thrombectomy, or removal of thrombus, is done to decrease thrombus burden, limit distal embolization, and improve perfusion of the myocardium. It can be done manually or mechanically.

Manual Aspiration Catheters

- Dual lumen catheter that is passed over the guidewire and through the guiding catheter to the area of thrombus.
- Examples include the Export (Medtronic), Fetch (Boston Scientific), and Pronto (Vascular Solutions) catheters.
- Manual suction is applied using a large syringe and thrombus is aspirated.
- Several passes can be done to remove visual thrombus.

Mechanical Aspiration

- Indicated for lesions with thrombus and saphenous vein grafts SVGs).
- Available as the Angiojet (MEDRAD, Inc.).
- Creates a strong suction and removes thrombus mechanically via an aspiration catheter.
- Significant bradycardia can occur. Consider placement of a temporary pacemaker, especially for procedures involving the RCA or dominant LCx.

Distal Protection Devices

- Prevent embolization of thrombus and debris during PCI.
- Used primarily with SVG interventions.
- Types include distal filtration, distal balloon occlusion, and proximal occlusion devices.
- Examples include FilterWire EX/EZ (Boston Scientific), GuardWire (Medtronic), and Proxis (St. Jude Medical).

SPECIAL CIRCUMSTANCES IN PCI

ST-Segment Elevation Myocardial Infarction

STEMI is typically caused by the abrupt rupture of a plaque that creates a potent stimulus for platelet aggregation and thrombus formation, resulting in the sudden occlusion of an artery with thrombus. The myocardium supplied by the artery becomes ischemic and the patient develops chest pain and the characteristic electrocardiographic findings of STEMI. Blood flow needs to be rapidly reestablished. There are two primary strategies for patients presenting with STEMI: thrombolytics and primary PCI.

Essential Facts

Primary PCI is superior to thrombolytic therapy in reducing death, reinfarction, intracranial bleeding, reocclusion of the culprit vessel, and myocardial ischemia in STEMI patients. Shorter reperfusion times are consistently associated with lower in-hospital and 6-month mortality rates.

- In hospitals without a PCI-capable cath lab and when transfer to a hospital with these services cannot be done in a timely manner, a thrombolytic agent should be given within 30 minutes of the patient's arrival.
- For hospitals with PCI-capable cath lab, primary PCI is indicated. The goal for this therapy, often referred to as door to balloon time (D2B) or door to reperfusion time, is 90 minutes or less for presentation to the hospital to open vessel.
- When transfer to another hospital is required for primary PCI, the goal is within 120 minutes of presentation.

PCI in acute MI can be challenging. Routine aspiration thrombectomy prior to stent placement is no longer recommended.

Thrombolytic therapy, also referred to as fibrinolytic therapy, remains a recommendation for patients presenting with STEMI to hospitals that do not have an interventional cath lab. Most commonly, these agents are given in the emergency department to lyse the thrombus. Patients should receive a loading dose of aspirin (162 mg–325 mg). Concurrent heparin administration for at least 48 hours is recommended due to the thrombin-mediated prothrombotic state created by thrombolytics.

If a thrombolytic agent does not restore flow, patients will commonly be transferred to another hospital capable of PCI. If you work in a larger hospital that routinely receives patients in transfer from outlying areas, you will care for patients who have received thrombolysis. You may also administer thrombolytic agents if you do complex peripheral procedures that require thrombolytic infusions (Table 10.5).

Table 10.5

Thrombolytic/Fibrinolytic Agents

	Typical Dosing	Nursing Implications
Tenecteplase (TNKase)	For STEMI: Weight-based single bolus. 30 mg IV if 90 kg 30 mg IV if <60 kg 35 mg IV if 60–70 kg 40 mg IV if 70–80 kg 45 mg IV if 80–90 kg 50 mg IV if >90 kg	Patients should receive a loading dose of aspirin (162–325 mg). Concurrent heparin administration for at least 48 hours is recommended because of the thrombin-mediated pro-thrombotic state created by thrombolytics. Bleeding is the most common adverse effect of all thrombolytic agents.
Alteplase (Ativase) tPA	For STEMI: Weight based. Infuse 15 mg over 1–2 minutes, then 50 mg over 30 minutes, and then remaining amount over 30 minutes (for weight >67 kg).	
Reteplace (Reteplase) r-PA	For STEMI: 10 unit IV bolus over 2 minutes followed by an additional 10 unit bolus over 2 minutes, 30 minutes after the first bolus.	

STEMI, ST-segment elevation myocardial infarction.

Saphenous Vein Grafts

SVG intervention can be challenging because of the nature of the vein graft. No reflow can be a significant complication. It is common to use embolic protection devices during SVG intervention to collect the debris. PCI for SVGs is associated with suboptimal results due to high rates of periprocedural MI and high rates of restenosis requiring target lesion revascularization (TLR).

Left Main Disease

Left main (LM) disease is rare in patients presenting with ACS. In the GRACE registry, the incidence was about 4%. Patients with acute MI and an LM culprit are more frequently in cardiogenic shock and are more likely to have had prehospital cardiac arrest compared to patients without an LM culprit. LM PCI can be technically difficult and is typically considered a high-risk procedure. In a "protected" LM, there is at least one patent bypass graft to the LCx or left anterior descending (LAD) artery or collateral flow. An unprotected LM lesion does not have this.

Key points to remember when assisting with LM PCI:

- Hemodynamic support may be initiated before PCI, especially if the patient has decreased LV function. Support may be from intra-aortic balloon pump or a percutaneous ventricular assist device such as Impella.
- Physicians should avoid placing guiding catheter too deeply into the ostium.
- Intravascular ultrasound (IVUS) guidance can be helpful.

Bifurcation Lesions

Bifurcations are vulnerable to plaque development because of blood flow, turbulence, and shear stress. Historically, PCIs of bifurcation lesions have had a lower success rate and increased MACE and they remain a challenge in PCI today. The cardiologist must consider the location of the diseased bifurcation as well as the size of the side branch. Two guidewires are used with one placed in the main branch and the other in the side branch. The use of DES is recommended.

- The provisional stenting technique is often done for bifurcation lesions. One stent is placed in the main artery and a second stent is placed in the side branch only if needed for dissection or impaired flow.

- Additional complex approaches to bifurcation stenting include the T technique, T stenting and small protrusion (TAP), reverse crush, culotte, mini-crush, and double kissing crush.
- A stent made specifically for bifurcation lesions is now available in the United States. The cobalt-chromium Tryton Side Branch stent (Tryton Medical) is deployed in the side branch. A DES is then inserted through it into the main artery and is deployed.

Chronic Total Occlusions

A chronic total occlusion (CTO) is a 100% high-grade native coronary stenosis with thrombolysis in myocardial infarction (TIMI) grade 0 flow, typically of at least 3 months' duration. Patients with CTOs may benefit from undergoing PCI as opening a CTO can reduce angina and decrease the need for coronary artery bypass grafting (CABG) surgery. CTO lesions are typically very complex and can be challenging to complete. Antegrade crossing of the CTO can be done; some cases may also require a retrograde approach where the lesion is approached from the collaterals. It can be very difficult to advance the guidewire through the occlusion and remain in the true lumen of the artery. Physician skill and patience are needed for wiring collaterals, retrograde wire tracking, and using special subintimal luminal reentry systems. Many CTO procedures require multiple guidewires, specialized catheters, and multiple stents. Guidewires for CTO procedures are stiffer at the tip and may have a hydrophilic coating.

SUMMARY

Catheter-based intervention as primary treatment of coronary artery disease (CAD) has experienced tremendous growth over the past 30 years. The overall complication rate of PCI has decreased significantly and now the mortality rate and the need for emergency bypass surgery is less than 1.0%. The ability to anticipate and intervene quickly and competently during PCI is essential.

11

Adjunctive Modalities

The most commonly used method to describe coronary artery disease continues to be coronary angiography. It is well known, however, that angiography does not always tell the whole story of the degree and extent of disease. Angiography is two-dimensional and does not provide functional information about a lesion or detailed information about the vessel wall. Fractional flow reserve (FFR) and instantaneous wave-free (iFR) ratio are available to provide physiological and functional data about the severity of a lesion. Intravascular ultrasound and optical coherence tomography (OCT) are available for enhanced imaging details inside the vessels.

In this chapter, you will learn:

1. When to use FFR
2. How to induce hyperemia
3. When to use iFR ratio
4. When to use intravascular ultrasound during stenting
5. Advantages of OCT

FRACTIONAL FLOW RESERVE

FFR is a physiological assessment of the coronary blood flow across a lesion during maximal hyperemia or stress, using a special guidewire-based product. It is helpful in determining if a lesion is

Table 11.1

Medications Used to Induce Hyperemia

	Typical Dosing	Nursing Implications
Adenosine IV	140 mcg/kg/min	■ Less than 2 minutes to maximal hyperemia. ■ Decreases BP 10%–15%. ■ Can cause chest burning, shortness of breath, flushing, and bronchospasm.
Adenosine IC	50–120 mcg LCA 30–60 mcg RCA	■ Short half-life; back to baseline within 60 seconds. ■ Transient heart block when injected into dominant coronary artery. ■ Less systemic effect than with IV adenosine.
Dobutamine IV	20–40 mcg/kg/min	■ Causes tachycardia, increases blood pressure.
Nitroprusside IC	0.3–0.9 mcg	■ Causes lowering of BP.
Regadenosan IV	0.4 mg	■ Causes tachycardia.

BP, blood pressure; IC, intracoronary; LCA, left coronary artery;
RCA, right coronary artery.

significant. FFR is the measured ratio of the mean distal coronary pressure divided by the mean proximal aortic pressure during maximal hyperemia. The normal FFR ratio is 1.0. Lesions with a measured FFR less than 0.8 are considered significant. Hyperemia is generally induced with adenosine; however, other agents can be used. See Table 11.1 for dosing guidelines.

FFR is useful because angiography is two-dimensional and cannot always demonstrate the clinical significance of a lesion and lesion treatment should be based on the presence of ischemia. The patient should be anticoagulated prior to advancing the 0.014 inch (0.035 cm) guidewire with high-fidelity transducer mounted 1.5 cm from the tip to measure FFR. A dose of nitroglycerin may be given intracoronary (IC) before the FFR guidewire is passed. The guidewire is advanced past the lesion and hyperemia is induced. Mean and phasic pressures are recorded, and at peak hyperemia, the FFR is calculated. FFR has been found to be superior to intravascular ultrasound (IVUS) for assessing the hemodynamic impact of a lesion.

INSTANTANEOUS WAVE-FREE RATIO

IFR pressure assesses stenosis severity at rest. It measures the ratio of distal coronary pressure to the aortic pressure during an isolated period during diastole, called the "wave-free period." Hyperemia is not needed, so no adenosine is administered. The normal iFR value is 1.0; findings below 0.9 suggest flow restriction.

Essential Facts

In FFR, a finding less than or equal to 0.80 is considered significant.

In iFR, a finding less than or equal to 0.90 is considered significant.

INTRAVASCULAR ULTRASOUND

IVUS is used as an adjunct in percutaneous coronary intervention (PCI) to image coronary arteries and stent deployment from within the vessel. It can differentiate between plaque and luminal irregularities and dissections. IVUS can be helpful in assessing vessel size, plaque morphology, and in-stent restenosis, and stent apposition.

There are two types of ultrasound: mechanical and phased array. In mechanical ultrasound, there is one rotating miniaturized transducer located at the tip of catheter, while in phased array, several transducers are present. Reflected ultrasound waves are used to provide images.

Imaging catheters are 3 Fr to 3.5 Fr in diameter and can be used within 5 Fr or 6 Fr guiding catheters. Before imaging, heparin should be given to obtain ACT greater than 250 seconds. Nitroglycerin may be given to induce maximal vasodilation and prevent spasm. The IVUS catheter is advanced over the guidewire. The distal end of the catheter is placed beyond the area to be imaged and is then pulled back through the area of stenosis. The IVUS catheter can be manually pulled back or mounted on automatic pull-back device that moves it along the arterial segment at a known and constant speed. The catheter quickly rotates to obtain cross-sectional images.

OPTICAL COHERENCE TOMOGRAPHY

OCT relies on backscattering (reflection) of light wavelength to obtain cross-sectional views. OCT allows for detailed characterization of morphological features of coronary arteries, plaques, and stents. It has higher resolution images than IVUS. It creates cross-sectional images of the coronary artery wall, which appears as a circular structure with three concentric layers.

OCT has a higher accuracy to detect early atherosclerosis, necrotic core, or lipid-rich tissues and a higher accuracy to detect thrombus and allows for visualization of calcification without blooming artifact. Thrombi are seen as masses protruding into the lumen discontinuous from the surface of the vessel wall. OCT is highly sensitive in diagnosing intracoronary thrombus.

OCT requires a blood-free zone for imaging, as blood scatters the OCT signal. It cannot be used to assess ostial lesion, as it is difficult to clear blood. It can cause ischemia due to the need for blood displacement. Anticoagulation is needed prior to placement to prevent thrombus formation. Nitroglycerin may be given to decrease the risk of coronary spasm. Some cardiologists may place the patient on 2 weeks of dual antiplatelet therapy (DAPT) following OCT, as endothelial damage has been found in animal studies.

Potential complications include dissection and ventricular fibrillation due to occlusion. Transient ischemia can occur, causing chest pain and ST segment changes. Careful attention to flushing, contrast injection, and wire management is needed, as there is a risk for air embolism.

SUMMARY

Additional tools that can be used during coronary angiography and PCI include physiological assessment such as FFR and iFR. If more information is needed about potential dissection or the adequacy of stent deployment, IVUS and OCT can be performed. If you work in a cath lab with these modalities available, be sure you are familiar with how to prepare and connect the catheters.

12

Procedural Complications

Thousands of cath procedures are performed daily in the United States and worldwide. Cath lab procedures, in general, are safe and the overall complication rate is low. Major complications, which occur rarely, include myocardial infarction (MI), stroke, and death. The most common procedural complications are related to access and include bleeding, hematoma, and vascular injury. These are reviewed in Chapter 5. This chapter reviews the remaining potential complications of cath lab procedures and outlines key interventions.

In this chapter, you will learn:

1. Patients at higher risk of developing complications
2. Potential complications of cath lab procedures
3. Tips for the early identification of complications
4. Interventions for various complications
5. When a cath patient may need to go to surgery

HIGH-RISK PATIENTS

Patients at higher risk for complications during cath lab procedures include those with the following signs:

- Left ventricular (LV) dysfunction
- Advanced age

- Triple vessel coronary disease
- Aortic stenosis

Other factors that can increase the risk to patients include coagulopathies, severe renal insufficiency, and severe peripheral arterial disease.

POTENTIAL COMPLICATIONS OF CATH LAB PROCEDURES

Many of the complications discussed in this chapter can occur in both diagnostic procedures and percutaneous coronary interventional procedures.

Arrhythmias

Minor arrhythmias and premature ventricular contractions (PVCs) can occur frequently during cath lab procedures and do not require treatment. Major arrhythmias—including significant bradycardia, heart block, ventricular tachycardia, ventricular fibrillation (VF), and asystole—may also occur during cath lab procedures and treatment or intervention may quickly be needed.

- Bradycardia may occur during coronary angiography, especially during the injection of the right coronary artery (RCA). Depending on the rate and the duration of the bradycardia, treatment may not be indicated. Asking the patient to cough, which increases intrathoracic pressure, may be all that is needed to restore normal rhythm. If the bradycardia is sustained, atropine and a temporary pacemaker may be needed. For some procedures involving a dominant RCA or left circumflex (LCx), a temporary pacemaker wire may be prophylactically placed to ensure back-up pacing during the procedure.
- A temporary pacing wire may be placed when a patient has a preexisting left bundle branch block (LBBB) when a right heart catheterization is planned. If the pulmonary artery (PA) catheter touches the area of the right bundle on the septum during advancement, and the left bundle branch is already blocked, the patient can develop asystole.
- Supraventricular tachycardia during procedures is not common. Treatment consists of potential vagal maneuvers or IV beta-blockers or calcium channel blockers. If the patient is hemodynamically unstable due the rapid heart rate, the patient may need synchronized cardioversion.
- Ventricular arrhythmias may be catheter induced, for example, when the pigtail is advanced into the LV. PVCs and ventricular

tachycardia due to catheter placement are usually self-limiting and respond well to repositioning of the catheter, and the administration of an anti-arrhythmic drug such as lidocaine is generally not needed. VF can follow the injection of the conus branch of the RCA or a nondominant RCA.

- Sustained ventricular tachycardia or VF can occur, especially in a patient with significant MI. Treatment with amiodarone 300 mg IV or lidocaine 50 mg to 75 mg IV and/or cardioversion/ defibrillation may be needed. Initiate cardiopulmonary support (CPR) and other resuscitative measures as needed.

Vasovagal Reactions

- Caused by stimulation of the vagal nerve, which causes parasympathetic nervous system stimulation.
- Signs and symptoms can include bradycardia, hypotension, pallor, diaphoresis, nausea, and yawning.
- Triggered by pain, anxiety, and/or a full bladder.
- Can occur while obtaining arterial access and during postprocedure sheath removal.
- The elderly may have hypotension without bradycardia.
- Can be poorly tolerated if the patient has underlying significant aortic stenosis.
- Vagal stimulation is one of earliest findings in cardiac perforation, as the pericardium is irritated by blood causing discomfort.
- Treat with atropine and normal saline boluses; elevate the patient's legs to promote venous return.
- Rarely, vasoactive drugs may be needed.

Contrast Allergy and Contrast-Induced Acute Kidney Injury

This topic is reviewed in Chapter 3.

Hypotension

There can be many reasons for hypotension during procedures. Causes of hypotension during procedures may include:

- Vasovagal stimulation
- Bleeding
- Poor cardiac output
- Contrast reaction
- Myocardial ischemia
- Cardiac tamponade

Right heart catheterization may be helpful in determining the underlying cause of hypotension.

Flash Pulmonary Edema

Sudden respiratory distress due to LV failure, leading to pulmonary edema, can occur during cardiac cath procedures. Treatment includes:

- Elevate head and upper body using wedge
- Oxygen administration
- Diuretics, nitrates, morphine
- Intubation and mechanical ventilation may be indicated
- Unloading LV with intra-aortic balloon counterpulsation or percutaneous ventricular assist device

Stroke

Stroke is a dreaded complication of cath procedures and is most commonly caused by an emboli, which can be air, thrombus, or aortic plaque. Extensive aortic atherosclerosis, commonly referred to as porcelain aorta, greatly increases the risk of stroke during cath lab procedures. Treatment of acute stroke during or immediately after cardiac cath procedures depends on the cause.

- Anticoagulation is indicated for thrombotic stroke; neurointervention and/or the administration of tissue plasminogen activator (tPA) may also be indicated.
- Rapid neurological assessment followed by CT scanning is indicated.
- Many hospitals have established stroke protocols that can be activated when a patient develops new signs and symptoms of stroke. Be familiar with stroke protocols at your facility.

Aortic Root Dissection

Catheter-induced dissection of the aorta is a rare but serious procedural complication.

- Class I: Dissection involves the ipsilateral cusp.
- Class II: Dissection involves the cusp and extends up the aorta less than 40 mm.
- Class II: Dissection involves the cusp and extends up the aorta greater than 40 mm.
- Class I and Class II aortic dissections are typically stented and the systolic blood pressure is carefully controlled. A follow-up transesophageal echocardiography (TEE) or CT may be done to assess healing. Class III aortic dissections generally require surgical correction.

Perforation of the Heart or Great Vessels

This is a rare but serious complication associated with procedures where stiffer catheters and wires may be used, such as transseptal catheterization, right ventricular biopsy, valvuloplasty, and pacemaker wire insertion. Perforation of the heart can lead to cardiac tamponade, caused by blood in the pericardial space.

Pericardial Effusion and Tamponade

Pericardial effusion is the presence of fluid in the pericardial space. Fluid collects in the pericardial space, exerting pressure on the heart. Echocardiography may be done to confirm the diagnosis. A pericardiocentesis may be needed to drain the fluid. See Chapter 15 for additional information.

Essential Facts

Classic clinical findings in cardiac tamponade include tachycardia, hypotension, elevated jugular venous pressure, pulsus paradoxus, and distant heart sounds.

Air Embolism

Air embolism is a rare but preventable complication of coronary angiography (Figure 12.1). Its reported incidence is less than 0.3% but it is likely underreported. It can be caused by inadequate aspiration

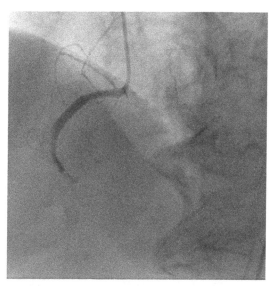

Figure 12.1 Air embolism in the right coronary artery.

of air and/or flushing of the catheter or pressure tubings, a defective manifold, or a balloon rupture. It can also occur during catheter exchanges when the hemostatic valve is left open. Symptoms depend on the amount of air that is introduced. Bubbles can sometimes be seen in the coronaries. Patients may have chest pain with or without ST segment elevation, hypotension, and arrhythmias. MI, no reflow, slow flow, and cardiac arrest can occur.

Essential Facts

To treat air embolism, perform the following:

- Initiate 100% oxygen per mask to dissipate the bubbles.
- Consider catheter aspiration; dissipate air with a wire or balloon or by forceful injection of saline.
- Treat no flow with adenosine, verapamil, or nitroprusside.
  - Give analgesics for chest pain.
  - Anticipate aggressive hemodynamic support: fluids, vasopressors, treatment of arrhythmias, and mechanical support.

The addition of performing percutaneous coronary intervention (PCI) brings additional risks and potential complications. Major complications of PCI include abrupt closure, major dissection, perforation, and no-reflow phenomenon. All can cause myocardial ischemia, leading to MI and possible death. The ability to quickly recognize and intervene appropriately when these complications occur is crucial.

Abrupt Closure

The abrupt obstruction of flow is often due to dissection with medial injury and the development of thrombus. It is a serious complication associated with death, MI, and the need for surgery. The patient develops ischemic pain and ST segment changes on the ECG and may become hypotensive and bradycardic. For patients who have severe hemodynamic instability, vasoactive and inotropic agents may be needed as well as the placement of an intra-aortic balloon catheter or a short-term ventricular assist device.

Prompt reintervention should be done to reestablish antegrade flow and thrombectomy may be required. Intravascular ultrasound may be useful to assess for dissection and for proper stent apposition and expansion. Additional anticoagulation is needed and the use of a glycoprotein IIb/IIIa receptor blocker should be considered. Consider $P2Y_{12}$ resistance in patients treated with clopidogrel. Once

Table 12.1

Coronary Artery Dissection Types	
Type A	Dissection with minor radiolucent areas, luminal haziness within the lumen without reduced flow
Type B	Little to no contrast in the presence of a parallel track or double lumen separated by a radiolucent area during contrast injection
Type C	Persistent extraluminal contrast staining after injection
Type D	Spiral dissection
Type E	Dissection with new and filling defects, reduce flow
Type F	Total occlusion of flow

Source: From Moscucci, M. (2013). *Grossman and Baim's cardiac catheterization, angiography, and intervention* (8th ed.). Philadelphia, PA: Lippincott, Williams, and Wilkins; Topol, E. J., & Teirstein, P.S. (Ed.). (2016). *Textbook of interventional cardiology.* Philadelphia, PA: Elsevier.

the patient has stabilized, more potent antiplatelet therapy should be considered.

Coronary Artery Dissection

The injection of contrast when the tip of the coronary catheter is against the arterial wall can cause a dissection, or split or tear, in the intimal or the medial layers of the artery. Dissections can also be caused by guiding catheters, guidewires, and devices or may be due to the "controlled injury" that is associated with balloon angioplasty. A classification system exists for coronary artery dissection types. See Table 12.1 for additional information.

Depending upon the extent of the dissection, patients can develop chest pain and ST segment changes. Larger dissections can lead to abrupt closure, MI, closure of major side branches, and cardiac tamponade. Small, focal dissections respond well to stenting while extensive dissection may not be completely treatable with stents. If untreated, it is associated with increased risk of MI, side branch closure, perforation and tamponade, and mortality. The inability to stent an extensive dissection in a major artery remains a reason for surgery.

Treatment depends on the extent of the perforation. A Type I perforation usually responds well to a prolonged balloon inflation.

Coronary Artery Perforation

A perforation occurs when the intimal, medial, and adventitial walls of the coronary artery are disrupted and there is extravasation of

Table 12.2

Classification of Coronary Perforation	
I	No extravasation
II	Pericardial or myocardial blush/staining
II	Perforation >1 mm with contrast streaming or cavity spilling, high risk for tamponade
Cavity spilling	Perforation into an anatomic chamber, coronary sinus

Source: From Moscucci, M. (2013). *Grossman and Baim's cardiac catheterization, angiography, and intervention* (8th ed.). Philadelphia, PA: Lippincott, Williams, and Wilkins; Topol, E. J., & Teirstein, P. S. (Ed.). (2016). *Textbook of interventional cardiology*. Philadelphia, PA: Elsevier.

blood. It can be caused by trauma from a stiff or hydrophilic guidewire, cutting balloon, atherectomy device, laser catheter, and so forth. See Table 12.2 for classifications of coronary artery perforations. Freely extravastating contrast is a true emergency. A prolonged balloon inflation (several minutes) should be done to see if that will stop the bleeding. If not, anticoagulation should be reversed. If the patient develops signs and symptoms of tamponade, set up for pericardiocentesis. The placement of a covered stent may be indicated. A cardiothoracic surgeon may be consulted.

No-Reflow Phenomenon

The no-reflow phenomenon is the acute cessation of antegrade blood flow in the coronary artery without evidence of physical obstruction, such as dissection, vasospasm, or air embolism. The underlying pathophysiology is not clearly understood but it is thought to be a result of distal embolization of thrombus and vasospasm. There is a higher incidence in acute MI, thrombus containing lesion, rotational atherectomy, and saphenous vein graft (SVG) intervention. When planning an intervention on a SVG, a distal protection device should be used. During an episode of no reflow, patients can become very unstable. They may develop chest pain, arrhythmias, and hemodynamic compromise. No reflow is associated with higher rates of MI and death.

Treatment of no-reflow phenomenon includes:

- Administration of nitroprusside, nicardipine, adenosine, verapamil, and/or diltiazem.
- Give through the angioplasty balloon to ensure medications reach the distal coronary bed.

- Consider use of IV glycoprotein IIb/IIIa receptor inhibitor.
- Additional hemodynamic support may be needed.
- Maintain activated clotting time (ACT) greater than 250 seconds.

Myocardial Ischemia and Infarction

MI is a known complication of PCI. Causes may include side-branch occlusion, no reflow phenomenon, prolonged balloon inflations, and hypotension. It is likely underreported, as biomarker measurement may not routinely be done. Ischemic chest pain within 48 hours following stenting is usually procedure related due to progression of dissection, side branch occlusion, slow flow, no reflow, coronary perforation, prolonged hypotension, or distal embolization.

Retained Equipment

While uncommon, equipment failures can occur. Wires can become entrapped or break. These failures can lead to occlusion of the artery. Removal should be done if possible. Snares, bioptomes, or baskets may be needed to remove retained equipment and wire fragments. If unable to be removed, this may be a reportable event, depending on your state regulations and hospital policies.

Nonischemic Chest Pain

Chest pain without an apparent cause is also seen. The pain is often atypical or pleuritic in nature and occurs within the first 24 hours of procedure. There are no ECG or biomarker changes. It is thought to be due to the stretching and overdilation of the arterial wall. It is commonly referred to as stretch pain. It must be carefully assessed to differentiate it from ischemic pain.

SUMMARY

Overall, cardiac catheterization and PCI are safe procedures; however, as with any procedure, complications can occur. The more common complications have been reviewed, interventions discussed, and implications for nursing care outlined. Early recognition and prompt treatment is essential to good patient outcomes.

13

Peripheral Angiography and Intervention

Atherosclerosis is a systemic disease and it is common for patients with significant coronary artery disease to also have peripheral arterial disease (PAD). PAD is more prevalent in our aging population and impacts quality of life. Noncoronary or peripheral angiography and intervention is increasingly being done in cath labs. This chapter reviews key points for angiography of the cerebrovascular system, the carotids, the renals, the aortoiliac system, and the lower extremities.

In this chapter, you will learn:

1. Normal and bovine aortic arch anatomy
2. How carotid stenting is done
3. When renal intervention can be beneficial
4. Indications for lower extremity intervention
5. The six Ps of acute limb ischemia (ALI)

GENERAL PRINCIPLES

- Peripheral angiography requires a larger image intensifier (12 inches–15 inches [30 cm–37.5 cm]) than coronary angiography (9 inches [22.5 cm]) to provide a larger field of view.

- Digital subtraction angiography (DSA) is the preferred imaging modality for peripheral angiography. Road-mapping software may be used with imaging.
- Femoral arterial access may need to be antegrade rather than retrograde for intervention of lower extremities.

CAROTID ANGIOGRAPHY AND INTERVENTION

Anatomy Review

- In the majority of the population, the arch of the aorta has three branches:
  - Brachiocephalic artery, also referred to as the innominate artery (which divides into right common carotid artery and the right subclavian artery)
  - Left common carotid artery
  - Left subclavian artery
- Variants of the aortic arch can be seen. See Figure 13.1. The most common variant is referred to as a *bovine arch* and it occurs in about 20% of the population. In a bovine arch, the brachiocephalic (innominate) artery shares a common origin with the left common carotid artery.

The proximal internal carotid artery and the bifurcation of the carotid artery can be affected by atherosclerotic changes that may lead to neurological changes such as transient ischemic attacks or stroke. For select patients, carotid intervention may be appropriate, especially those who are poor surgical candidates.

Indications for carotid intervention include symptomatic or asymptomatic high-grade stenosis of the internal carotid artery. Intervention is contraindicated if visible thrombus is present or if there is an active infection.

Careful evaluation of the aortic arch is needed prior to carotid intervention. If bilateral carotid stenosis is present, the procedures should be staged or done at separate times. Baseline angiography of the anterior cerebral circulation is recommended prior to intervention. Perform a full neurological assessment using the National Institutes of Health Stroke Scale.

Prior to intervention, the patient should be pretreated with dual antiplatelet therapy (DAPT). Antibiotic prophylaxis may be indicated. Light procedural sedation is generally preferred to allow monitoring of the patient's neurological status. Femoral access is most commonly used. Administer heparin (bivalirudin has been used) and maintain activated clotting time (ACT) between 200 second and 250 seconds.

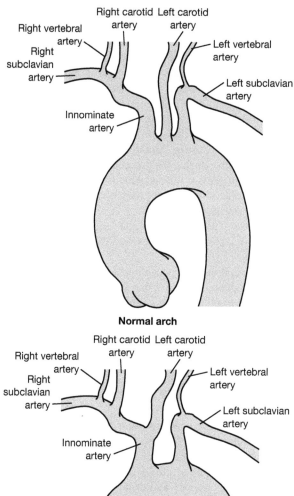

Figure 13.1 Aortic arch and bovine arch.

The use of a cerebral protection device is recommended to decrease the risk of stroke. Retrograde flow devices may be incorporated into the procedure. Perform angiography of the anterior cerebral circulation after the balloon and the cerebral protection device are removed, to compare to the baseline images. Predilation of the stenosis may be needed prior to stent placement. Be prepared to administer atropine in the event of bradycardia. Self-expanding stents are typically used. Tapered carotid stents are available in 6 mm to 9 mm diameter and 30 mm to 40 mm in length. Drug-eluting stents (DES) are usually not needed because of the low rate of restenosis following carotid intervention.

Whenever possible during the procedure, perform a quick neurological assessment. This can be accomplished by placing a squeaky toy in the contralateral hand. Have the patient squeeze it when asked to assess extremity movement.

Following stent deployment, repeat angiography to document final results and compare to previous images to exclude distal embolization.

Potential complications of carotid intervention include slow flow, hypotension and bradycardia caused by baroreceptor stretching when near the carotid sinus, and stroke. Hyperperfusion syndrome is a rare but potentially life-threatening complication.

Post procedure, lifelong aspirin and an oral antiplatelet agent for at least 30 days are recommended.

RENAL ANGIOGRAPHY AND INTERVENTION

Some patients with severe hypertension (<5%) have renal artery stenosis (RAS) and may benefit from renal intervention. The stenosis can be unilateral or bilateral. RAS can be caused by atherosclerosis or fibromuscular dysplasia (FMD). Atherosclerotic disease is more common in patients over 45 and usually involves the aortic orifice or the proximal portion of the renal artery. FMD is a noninflammatory, nonatherosclerotic disorder that leads to stenosis, occlusion, aneurysms, and tortuosity of arteries, especially the renal and the carotid arteries. It is more common in women. Multifocal FMD, which is more common, has a classic "string of beads" appearance in angiography.

Obtain an abdominal aortogram prior to selective renal artery angiography to look for high-grade ostial lesions, accessory renal arteries, and heavy calcification. The use of DSA is preferred. The angiogram is done in the left anterior oblique (LAO) 20° using a diagnostic pigtail catheter placed below the diaphragm. A volume of 20 mL to 25 mL of contrast over 2 seconds is delivered.

If the patient has bilateral RAS, staging the procedure should be considered. Prior to renal intervention, pretreat with aspirin and hydration as indicated.

Access obtained from the contralateral femoral artery provides the best guiding catheter support. Catheters commonly used to selectively engage the renal artery include Judkins right, renal double curve, or multipurpose. If the physician does not want to directly engage the ostium of the renal, a shuttle sheath may be placed just outside it.

Coronary guidewires are used but the use of hydrophilic wires is not recommended due to the risk of increased perforation. Anticoagulation is indicated and the ACT goal during the procedure is 250 seconds to 300 seconds.

Balloon angioplasty alone is often successful in FMD. Direct stenting is generally needed for patients with atherosclerotic RAS. Balloon expandable stents are used; sizes range from 4 mm to 6 mm × 12 mm to 18 mm. For ostial lesions, physicians will often "flare" the end of the stent in the aorta. Embolic protection devices may be used.

In addition to the complications related to arterial access, complications during and after renal intervention may include renal infarction, deterioration in renal function, distal embolization, dissection, cholesterol embolism, perforation, and thrombosis of the renal artery.

Post procedure, patients should receive DAPT for at least 30 days.

LOWER EXTREMITY PAD

Anatomy Review

- The aorta branches at the level of the fourth lumbar vertebra into the iliac arteries, which divide into internal and external branches.
- The internal iliac arteries supply the pelvic organs.
- The external iliac artery becomes the common femoral artery (CFA) below the inguinal ligament.
- The CFA bifurcates into the profunda femoris (deep femoral artery) and the superficial femoral artery (SFA).
- The SFA becomes the popliteal artery after it passes through the adductor canal above the knee.
- The popliteal artery trifurcates below the knee into the anterior tibial, peroneal, and posterior tibial arteries (Figure 13.2).

PAD of the lower extremities includes atherosclerotic disease of the aortoiliac, femoropopliteal, and infrapopliteal arterial segments. It is a commonly seen disease that affects over 200 million people internationally. PAD is associated with increased morbidity,

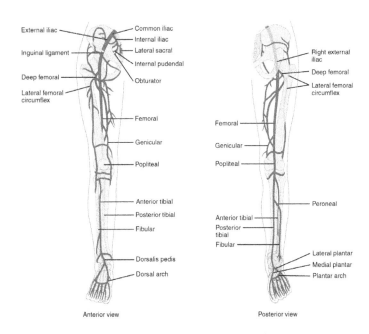

Anterior view

Posterior view

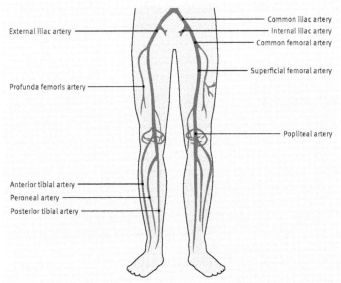

Figure 13.2 Lower extremity anatomy.

mortality, and decreased quality of life. Clinical findings suggestive of PAD include a history of claudication, impaired walking function, and ischemic rest pain. Patients may have poor pulses, vascular bruits, pallor, and nonhealing wounds, or gangrene.

Medical therapy for these patients includes lifestyle modification, structured exercise, smoking cessation, and medications such as antiplatelet agents and statins. Treatment of coexisting hypertension and diabetes is essential. Patients should be instructed to do regular examinations of their feet, monitoring for wounds and signs of infection.

Indications for intervention include symptom relief, management of chronic limb ischemia, and repair of complications related to other cath procedures. Interventional therapy to treat lower extremity PAD includes balloon angioplasty, stent placement, and atherectomy.

Essential Facts

- Critical limb ischemia (CLI) is chronic ischemic rest pain (longer than 2 weeks in duration), nonhealing wound/ulcers, or gangrene in one or both legs caused by PAD.
- ALI is characterized by the 6 Ps of severe limb hypoperfusion: pain, pallor, pulselessness, poikilothermia (cold), paresthesia, and paralysis of less than 2 weeks' duration. It is considered a medical emergency and the patient should be seen by a vascular surgeon.

Iliac Interventions

- Indicated for treatment of intermittent claudication not responding to medical therapy, CLI, and flow-limiting dissections following a cath procedure.
- DSA is considered the gold standard for imaging.
- Access is generally retrograde if the CFA is not involved or can be from the ipsilateral or the contralateral CFA.
- Both balloon-expanding and self-expanding stents can be used.
- Complication rates are low but access site bleeding, hematoma, retroperitoneal bleeding, and distal embolization can occur.
- Post procedure, life-time aspirin is needed as well as 30 days of an antiplatelet agent.

Femoropopliteal Interventions

- The SFA is a common site for stenosis or occlusion.
- Access can be from the contralateral CFA, the ipsilateral CFA, the brachial artery, or the popliteal artery.

- Balloon angioplasty may be done for short single lesions unless the SFA origin or the distal popliteal is not involved.
- Stenting may be considered. Several peripheral vascular bare metal stents are available. The drug-eluting Zilver PTX (Cook Medical) stent is approved for use in the SFA.
- Adjunctive modalities such as laser/orbital atherectomy or cutting balloon may be used.
- Drug-eluting balloons are also available.
- Procedural complications can include dissection, perforation, and distal embolization.

Infrapopliteal Interventions

- Indications for intervention include severe claudication, limb-threatening ischemia, limb salvage, and nonhealing wounds.
- The ipsilateral antegrade approach is useful for long occlusions, severe calcification, or distal disease. Access from the contralateral CFA using a crossover approach is common for proximal, focal disease.
- Atherectomy, stents, and drug-coated balloons may be used.
- Complications may include vasospasm, no reflow, thrombosis, perforation, and flow-limiting dissection.

SUMMARY

Increasingly, catheter-based techniques are being safely completed for atherosclerotic disease of the peripheral arterial system. Carotid and renal intervention will continue to evolve as technologies advance. More options will also be available for patients with symptomatic PAD to improve circulation, healing, and quality of life.

14

Structural Heart Procedures

Structural heart procedures or noncoronary artery interventions are increasingly common in cath labs, especially in larger centers. They require a fair amount of knowledge and expertise to be able to readily and competently assist. A basic overview of some of the structural heart procedures being done is provided in this chapter. For staff new to the cath lab, continue to hone and perfect your scrubbing techniques before jumping into these procedures, if possible.

In this chapter, you will learn:

1. Which structural heart procedures involve a transseptal puncture and approach
2. Procedures that can be done to close defects
3. When closure or occlusion of the left atrial appendage (LAA) might be indicated
4. Available options for catheter-based valve replacement and repair
5. When alcohol septal ablation may be recommended for hypertrophic cardiomyopathy

TRANSSEPTAL APPROACH

Several structural heart procedures require a transseptal approach to access the left heart. These procedures include septal defect closure, mitral repair and valvuloplasty, and LAA occlusion. The transseptal approach is detailed in Chapter 8. Risks associated with transseptal access include puncture of the aorta, the atrium, and stroke.

Essential Facts

Echocardiography monitoring via a transesophageal probe or an intracardiac catheter is commonly used as an adjunct in structural heart procedures to assist with sizing, positioning, and placement of the catheters, guidewires, closure devices, clips, and valves used in structural heart procedures.

DEFECT CLOSURES

Atrial Septal Defect Closure

Atrial septal defects (ASD) are a common congenital lesion and are classified into ostium primum, ostium secundum, sinus venosus, and coronary sinus types. Among the various types of ASDs, only the ostium secundum defect is amenable to catheter-based device closure. Indications for ASD closure include significant left-to-right shunting and cryptogenic stroke.

Approved devices include the Amplatzer Septal Occluder and the Gore HELEX septal occluder. Imaging with transesophageal or intracardiac echocardiography is needed. Angiography is done to outline the atrial anatomy. The ASD is crossed and a compliant sizing balloon is placed across it and inflated to determine the needed device size. The smallest size that covers the defect is chosen for placement.

Complications that can occur include device embolization or malposition, air embolism, perforation, residual shunting at the atrial level, infection, arrhythmias, thromboembolism, nickel allergy, and erosion. Endocarditis prophylaxis is recommended for 6 months following device placement.

Patent Foramen Ovale Closure

Patent foramen ovale (PFO) is a congenital tunnel-like passage in the interatrial septum lesion that can persist into adulthood. About 20% of the adult population have a PFO; it is not clear why it fails to close. Most patients are asymptomatic but a few may experience a crytogenic stroke, which is a stroke that may occur due to paradoxical embolism. PFO closure may be done for patients who have experienced a cryptogenic stroke as a way to prevent further stroke.

Examples of available devices include the Cardioform Septal Occluder (Gore) and the Amplatzer PFO Occluder. Imaging with ultrasound is needed during the closure procedure. Transseptal access is obtained and the PFO is crossed with a guidewire. Balloon size may be used to determine device size. The device is advanced into the left atrium (LA) and the left-sided occluder is opened and pulled back against the septum before the right-sided occluder is opened. After proper positioning is ensured, the device is released from the delivery system.

Complications that can occur include new-onset atrial fibrillation (AF), device migration and embolization, erosion, and device thrombosis.

LEFT ATRIAL APPENDAGE CLOSURE

The LAA has been identified as a major source for clot that embolizes and causes stroke in patients with chronic AF. Standard treatment of chronic AF is anticoagulation, but not all patients can tolerate anticoagulation. Catheter-based closure or occlusion of the LAA may be indicated for some patients who do not tolerate anticoagulation well, for example, patients with recurrent gastrointestinal bleeds, prior intracranial hemorrhage, or a history of falls with injury.

One currently approved device is the WATCHMAN (Boston Scientific). It is a self-expanding nitinol cage covered by a layer of polytetrafluoroethylene (PTFE). It is available in five sizes, ranging from 21 mm to 33 mm. Transesophageal echocardiography is performed to ensure there is no thrombus in the LA or LAA. The patient is anticoagulated with heparin. Transseptal access to the LA is then obtained. Positioning of the device within the atrial appendage is confirmed and the device is released and remains in place to occlude the orifice of the LAA.

Potential complications include vascular access site bleeding and hematoma, embolism of air or thrombus causing stroke, and cardiac tamponade. Embolization of the device can occur.

AORTIC VALVE INTERVENTIONS

Interventions currently approved for the treatment of aortic stenosis (AS) include aortic valvuloplasty and transcatheter aortic valve replacement (TAVR).

Aortic Valvuloplasty

Aortic valvuloplasty can be done for patients with symptomatic due to severe AS may be candidates for an aortic valvuloplasty as a short-term to TAVR or surgical aortic valve replacement. The goal of aortic valvuloplasty is to double the aortic valve area or decrease the gradient across the aortic valve by 50%.

After assessment of the aortic valve is done, a valvuloplasty balloon is placed across the valve and inflated. Rapid ventricular pacing (RVP) up to 220 beats/min may be done to lower the patient's blood pressure just prior to balloon inflation. Repeat inflations can be done as needed. If a large gradient continues, a larger balloon may be indicated.

Complications can include vascular access bleeding and hematoma, arrhythmias, ventricular perforation and tamponade, and embolic events causing stroke.

Transcatheter Aortic Valve Replacement

Many patients with AS who are poor surgical candidates may be considered for TAVR. The procedure may be done using sedation or general anesthesia. Approaches include the femoral artery (most common), subclavian artery, transapical, and transaortic. Currently available TAVR valves include the Sapien 3 (Edwards LifeSciences) and the CoreValve (Medtronic).

In many facilities, TAVR may be done by a team of cardiologists and cardiothoracic surgeons. The patient may be prepared ahead of time for conversion to open surgery if needed.

Complications of TAVR can include vascular access site bleeding and injury, heart block, and stroke.

Essential Facts

Some patients may need short-term pacing following the placement of the new valve, and some may require placement of a permanent pacemaker. Patients at higher risk of needing ongoing pacemaker support include those with preexisting first-degree heart block, right bundle branch block (RBBB), and left hemiblock.

MITRAL VALVE INTERVENTION

Interventions currently approved for the mitral valve include valvuloplasty for mitral stenosis and MitraClip for mitral regurgitation.

Mitral Valvuloplasty

Patients with untreated mitral stenosis, which is mostly caused by rheumatic fever, can develop significant symptoms including dyspnea, fatigue, pulmonary hypertension, and systemic embolization. Open surgical repair may be appropriate, while mitral valvuloplasty may be considered for patients who are thought to be poor surgical candidates.

Transseptal access to the mitral valve is obtained and a valvuloplasty balloon is placed across the stenotic mitral valve. The balloon is then inflated and deflated to separate the fused commissures of the mitral valve and relieve the degree of mitral stenosis.

Complications can include hypotension, arrhythmias, cardiac tamponade, and vascular access site bleeding.

MitraClip

Repair of degenerative mitral regurgitation using the catheter-based MitraClip is indicated for those patients with 3+ or 4+ mitral regurgitation who are failing maximal medical therapy to control their heart failure, have a prohibitive risk for surgical repair, and have anatomy that is amenable to clip placement. Patients with rheumatic mitral valve disease should not have this procedure.

Transseptal access to the mitral valve is obtained. Transesophageal echocardiography and fluoroscopy is used for imaging. A small clip is placed on the mitral valve leaflets to decrease the total size of the valve orifice and the amount of regurgitant flow.

Procedural complications can include access site bleeding, partial clip detachment, and device embolization (rare).

PARAVALVULAR LEAK REPAIR

A paravalvular leak is an uncommon complication of open valve repair. It occurs rarely following TAVR. Signs and symptoms include heart failure and hemolysis. A reoperation is usually not desired to repair the leak, as the risk is increased. Multiple catheter-based devices, occluders, and plugs are available to close a paravalvular leak in the cath lab. It is a technically challenging procedure. Careful imaging is important to procedural success.

ALCOHOL SEPTAL ABLATION FOR HYPERTROPHIC CARDIOMYOPATHY

In hypertrophic cardiomyopathy, the septal wall is markedly hypertrophic and there is diastolic dysfunction. It is a genetic autosomal dominant disease that impacts up to 1 in 500 people. Patients with this are at increased risk of arrhythmias, sudden cardiac death, angina, syncope, and heart failure.

Treatment options include medical management, dual chamber pacing, surgical septal myectomy, and alcohol septal ablation. In septal ablation, ethanol is introduced into the first or second septal branch of the left anterior descending (LAD) artery. The ethanol ablates the septal branch, inducing a myocardial infarction with resulting stunning and remodeling of the muscle. A temporary pacing wire is often placed, as transient heart block can occur. Prior to the instillation of the ethanol, careful assessment of the distal tip of the balloon is done to ensure no leaking of ethanol into the LAD.

Complications can include coronary artery dissection, complete heart block, and large myocardial infarction from errant ethanol injection. Up to 10% of patients may need a permanent pacemaker.

SUMMARY

This chapter has provided a basic review of some of the structural heart procedures being completed today. This will continue to be a growing field with rapidly changing technology. These procedures can be challenging to assist. Continue to grow your confidence and experience.

15

Emergency Care in the Cath Lab

While the majority of procedures done in the cath lab go well and are free of problems and complications, it is important to be able to recognize which patients are at a higher risk of decompensating during procedures. Situations you will learn to manage include bradycardia and other arrhythmias, hypotension, hypertension, and cardiac tamponade. Some patients will need immediate hemodynamic support. Knowing how to quickly and competently assist with the placement of an intra-aortic balloon catheter or short-term ventricular assist device is essential for improved patient outcome.

In this chapter, you will learn:

1. What patients are considered high risk during cardiac cath procedures
2. How bradycardia is managed
3. How hypotension is managed
4. The benefits of intra-aortic balloon counterpulsation
5. Which patients benefit from ventricular support devices

As noted in previous chapters, the patients at the highest risk for acute decompensation and poor outcomes during cardiac cath procedures include those with:

- Left ventricular (LV) dysfunction with ejection fraction less than 30%
- Acute myocardial infarction

- Cardiogenic shock
- Left main (LM) disease or multivessel coronary artery disease
- Severe aortic stenosis (AS)

MANAGING BRADYCARDIA

Causes of significant or prolonged bradycardia can include:

- Vasovagal reaction
- Heart block
- Right coronary artery occlusion

Pharmacologic agents, further described in Table 15.1, such as atropine and isoproterenol may be used for symptomatic bradycardia.

Temporary Pacing

Temporary pacing may be needed during procedures or as stand-alone therapy for patients with sustained bradycardia. Two different types of temporary pacemakers are commonly available in the cath lab setting: external transcutaneous pacing and transvenous pacing.

External Transcutaneous Pacing

Current defibrillators have the ability to provide external transcutaneous pacing. External pacing can be initiated quickly and it is useful

Table 15.1

Medications Used for Bradycardia

	Typical Dosing	Nursing Implications
Atropine	0.5–1 mg IV every 3–5 minutes as needed to max dose of 3 mg.	■ Anticholinergic drug that blocks parasympathetic stimulation. ■ Doses less than 0.5 mg can cause paradoxical bradycardia. ■ Potential adverse reactions include tachycardia, dry mouth, and urinary retention.
Isoproterenol (Isuprel)	1–10 mcg/min titrated for heart rate; rarely used for this outside of electrophysiology procedures and patients who have undergone cardiac transplantation.	■ For patients following heart transplantation due to denervation of the heart. ■ Positive inotropic and chronotropic effects. ■ Potential adverse reactions include tremor, tachycardia, and ventricular arrhythmias.

in an emergency setting when the patient abruptly develops severe bradycardia or asystole. To initiate external pacing, apply the combination pacing/defibrillation pad to the patient, in either an anterior or anterior-posterior placement. Connect the pads to the defibrillator, and activate the pacing mode of the defibrillator. Select the desired pacing rate and the pacing output in milliamperes (mA). For most adults, a rate of 70 beats to 80 beats per minute and an mA of 50 to 100 will provide a reliable capture of the ventricles. External pacing can be uncomfortable for the patient; treatment with analgesics or sedation may be needed for pacing. If sustained pacing is needed, transvenous placement of a pacing wire should be considered.

Temporary Transvenous Pacing

If the need for pacing is more sustained, transvenous pacing should be initiated. A pacing wire is placed through a venous sheath and advanced into the apex of the right ventricle. Some pacing wires are balloon directed and may be placed at the bedside. Fluoroscopy provides accurate placement of the pacing wire.

Equipment and supplies needed are:

- Temporary pacing wire, sheath
- Bridging cable
- Temporary pacemaker generator with new battery

Once placement in the right ventricular apex is completed and ventricular capture is confirmed, the *capture threshold*, measured in mA, should be determined. The *sensing threshold*, measured in millivolts (mV), can be assessed, unless the patient has significant bradycardia or is 100% dependent on the pacemaker.

- The capture threshold is the smallest amount of mA that is needed for capture. To determine the capture threshold, pace at a rate slightly faster than the patient's intrinsic rate to obtain 100% capture. While looking at the patient's rhythm on the monitor, slowly reduce the output (mA) until noncapture occurs. Increase the output until capture recurs. This mA value is the capture threshold. Set the pacemaker mA at two to three times the capture threshold.
- The sensing threshold indicates if the pacemaker is sensing the patient's own rhythm appropriately. Do not assess if the patient is dependent on the pacemaker or has an underlying significant bradycardia. To determine the sensing threshold, reduce the mA to its threshold (as determined in the preceding). While looking at the pacemaker generator, turn the sensitivity dial to a higher numerical setting until the sensing light stops. Then

turn the sensitivity dial toward the lower numerical setting until the sensitivity light begins flashing again. This is the sensitivity threshold. Set the pacemaker mV at half of the sensitivity threshold. Be certain to return the mA to its proper setting.

Complications of transvenous pacing include:

- Bleeding, hematoma at sheath insertion site
- Perforation of the atria or ventricle and cardiac tamponade
- Loss of capture or failure of sensing
- Pneumothorax/hemothorax with subclavian access

MANAGING HYPOTENSION

Hypotension can occur during procedures for several reasons. It is essential to identify the cause quickly so that the correct therapy can be determined and initiated. Factors than can cause hypotension during procedures include:

- Anaphylaxis
- Arrhythmias
- Cardiac tamponade
- Cardiogenic shock
- Drug effect
- Significant bleeding
- Vasovagal reaction

If it is unclear what is causing the hypotension, a right heart catheterization or stat transthoracic echo may be ordered to provide additional clinical information. Refer to Table 15.2 for additional information.

If the patient is experiencing a significant bleed, for example, a vascular perforation causing bleeding into the retroperitoneal space, anticipate orders for fluid boluses, including blood products and discontinuing anticoagulation, if possible. If cardiogenic shock is the cause of the hypotension, anticipate orders for inotropic and vasopressor agents. See Table 15.3 for medications that may be administered for hypotension.

MANAGING HYPERTENSION

High blood pressure can increase risks of bleeding, hematoma, and potential intracranial hemorrhage. You may be required to administer short-acting medications to lower a patient's blood pressure during

Table 15.2

Differentiating Causes of Hypotension

Hypovolemia	Cardiogenic	Vasodilation
↓RA, ↓PA, ↓CO, ↑SVR	↑RA, ↑PA, ↓CO, ↑SVR	↓RA, ↓PA, ↓CO, ↓SVR
■ Give saline boluses; blood transfusion may be needed. ■ May need temporizing vasopressors.	■ Assess for myocardial ischemia. ■ Provide vasopressors or possible circulatory support with intra-aortic balloon or short-term VAD.	■ Assess for vasovagal, excess nitrates, sedation/narcotic effect, and contrast reaction. ■ May need temporizing vasopressors. ■ May need treatment for anaphylactoid reaction.

CO, cardiac output; PA, pulmonary arterial pressure; RA, right atrial pressure; SVR, systemic vascular resistance; VAD, ventricular assist device.

Table 15.3

Medications That Raise Blood Pressure

	Typical Dosing	Nursing Implications
Dopamine	1–10 mcg/kg/min, continuous infusion.	■ Inotropic: increases contractility. ■ May increase HR. ■ At doses >10 mcg/kg/min, vasoconstriction and increased SVR occur. ■ Extravasation risk.
Norepinephrine (Levophed)	8–12 mcg/min, then titrate to effect, usually to maintain systolic BP of 80–100 mmHg. Usual maintenance dose is 2–4 mcg/min.	■ Potent vasoconstrictor. ■ Positive inotropic and positive chronotropic effects.
Phenylephrine (Neo-Syneprhine)	40–100 mcg IV every 1–2 minutes to maintain target BP; do not exceed 200 mcg. 0.5 mcg/kg/min, continuous infusion (max: 6 mcg/kg/min).	■ Potent vasoconstrictor. ■ Increases BP without increasing HR or contractility. ■ Reflex bradycardia may occur. ■ Extravasation risk.

BP, blood pressure; HR, heart rate; SVR, systemic vascular resistance.

Table 15.4

Medications for Hypertension

	Typical Dosing	Nursing Implications
Nitroglycerin	100–200 mcg IV bolus 5 mcg/min, increased by 5 mcg every 3–5 minutes for continuous IV infusion.	▪ One of the most commonly used drugs in the cath lab. ▪ Can be administered several ways: IV, IC, IA, SL. ▪ In addition to lowering BP, it is used for coronary spasm, to increase coronary blood flow, and to lower LVEDP.
Hydralazine (Apresoline)	5–20 mg IV bolus.	▪ Potent and direct arterial dilator. ▪ May cause a reflex tachycardia. ▪ Adverse effects include headache and nausea.
Metoprolol tartrate (Lopressor)	5 mg IV bolus every 2 minutes for three doses.	▪ May be used to manage BP in patients with an adequate HR. ▪ May be used in AMI patients who are hypertensive and tachycardic.
Enalprilat (Vasotec)	1.25–5 mg IV every 6 hours.	▪ Can worsen hyperkalemia.
Esmolol (Brevibloc)	80 mg bolus IV over 30 seconds, followed by a 150 mcg/kg/min IV infusion, if necessary.	▪ Ultra short-acting. ▪ Injection site reactions can occur. ▪ Can cause nausea.
Labetalol	20 mg IV over 2 minutes. Additional injections of 40 mg IV or 80 mg IV over 2 minutes may be administered in 10-minute intervals until the desired supine BP is achieved or a total of 300 mg is given.	▪ Contraindicated in patients with severe bradycardia or advanced heart block unless a functioning pacemaker is present.
Nicardipine (Cardene)	5 mg/hr to start.	▪ Use with care in AMI. ▪ Do not use in hypertrophic cardiomyopathy or aortic stenosis.
Nitroprusside (Nipride)	Start at 0.3 mcg/kg/min per continuous infusion, and titrate every 5 minutes until desired effect; max dose 10 mcg/kg/min.	▪ Potent arterial and venous dilator. ▪ May be given IC for marked vasospasm, no reflow. ▪ May be used in hypertensive crisis. ▪ Light sensitive, risk of cyanide toxicity with extended use.

AMI, acute myocardial infarction; BP, blood pressure; HR, heart rate; IA, intraarterial; IC, intracoronary; LVEDP, left ventricular end-diastolic pressure; SL, sublingual.

and immediately following procedures. See Table 15.4 for additional information about commonly used antihypertensive agents.

CARDIAC TAMPONADE

In cardiac tamponade, fluid (usually blood) collects in the pericardial space and compresses the heart. Classic signs and symptoms include tachycardia, hypotension, elevated jugular venous pressure, pulsus paradoxus, and distant heart sounds. The immediate treatment is pericardiocentesis and removal of the fluid.

Optimally, elevate the patient on a 30° to 45° wedge if possible. Echocardiography guidance may be requested. Most cardiologists use the subxiphoid approach. Prep and drape the patient. The cardiologist injects a local anesthetic. Using an 18G needle attached to a syringe partially filled with saline, they will advance the needle into the pericardial space. The syringe is disconnected and a 0.035 inch (0.09 cm) guidewire is advanced up into the pericardial space (Figure 15.1). The needle is removed and the catheter of choice is advanced into position over the guidewire. The guidewire is removed and the fluid/blood is removed. If the pericardial catheter is to remain in place, it is connected to a dependent drainage system. Sterile dressings are applied.

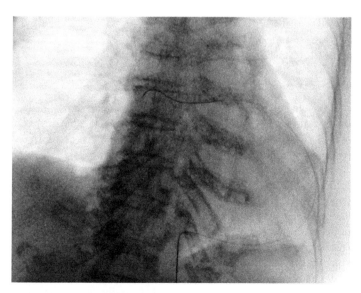

Figure 15.1 Wire in pericardial space.

MECHANICAL HEMODYNAMIC SUPPORT

Intra-Aortic Balloon Pumping

Essential Facts

Hemodynamic effects of intra-aortic balloon pump (IABP) therapy include increased coronary artery blood flow, decreased afterload, decreased preload, increased cardiac output, and decreased LV end-diastolic pressure.

Indications

- Cardiogenic shock
- Acute mitral regurgitation
- Acute ventricular septal defect
- Refractory chest pain
- Refractory ventricular arrhythmias
- Prophylaxis in patients with LM coronary disease pending surgery
- Weaning from cardiopulmonary bypass

Contraindications

- Aortic insufficiency (AI)
- Aortic dissection, abdominal aortic aneurysm
- Aortic stents
- Severe peripheral arterial disease

Developed in the late 1960s, the intra-aortic counterpulsation was the first method of cardiac support. There are several companies that make IABPs and catheters and it is important that you become very familiar with the type used at your facility.

The intra-aortic balloon catheter is a flexible dual lumen catheter with a long, large (30–50 mL) polyurethane balloon wrapped on it. One lumen delivers helium from the pump to the balloon; the second lumen allows passage of a guidewire and arterial pressure monitoring (Figure 15.2). The intra-aortic balloon catheter is placed percutaneously via the common femoral artery and advanced over the guidewire so that the distal tip of the balloon is below the subclavian artery and the proximal end is above the renal arteries. The catheter system is connected to a pump console that rapidly shuttles helium in and out of the balloon, synchronized with systole and diastole.

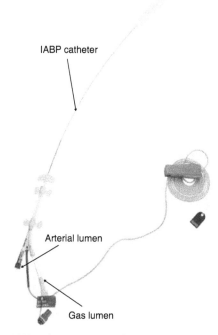

IABP catheter

Arterial lumen

Gas lumen

Figure 15.2 The IABP catheter connected to two lumens: arterial lumen and gas lumen.

IABP, intra-aortic balloon pump.

Source: Image courtesy of Teleflex Incorporated. © 2018 Teleflex Incorporated. All rights reserved. Retrieved from https://www.teleflex.com/usa/product-areas/interventional/cardiac-assist/intra-aortic-balloon-catheters/

Intra-aortic balloon counterpulsation can increase cardiac output by 10% to 20%. Recent data suggest that IABP therapy does not improve outcomes in cardiogenic shock and its use may be falling out of favor in some areas of the country.

Essential Facts

An intra-aortic balloon should *not* be used in a patient with AI. Counterpulsation will increase the volume of blood going back to the aortic arch and through the aortic valve during diastole and worsen the AI.

Trigger Modes

A trigger is required as a signal to the console to properly identify the cardiac cycle. Commonly used triggers include:

- ECG: Uses the R wave from the pump's leads that are placed prior to placement or from the cath lab monitor via a slave cable. This trigger is recommended for patients with arrhythmias or a pacemaker.
- Arterial pressure: Uses systolic upstroke of the arterial pressure waveform. Recommended with low-voltage R waves.
- Pacer: Used with paced rhythms.
- Automatic or internal: Used for pulseless rhythms, during cardiopulmonary support (CPR), and during cardiopulmonary bypass.

Insertion Techniques

- The femoral area is prepped and draped. Local anesthetic is administered.
- Using a modified Seldinger technique, the common femoral artery is cannulated with an 18G needle, and a 0.035 inch (0.09 cm) J-tipped guidewire is advanced through the needle after the brisk flow of arterial blood is confirmed.
- The guidewire should be advanced to the level of the descending aorta under fluoroscopic guidance.
- A small nick at the wire entry site is made to accommodate the sheath/catheter.
- The needle is removed and the arterial sheath is placed.
- The intra-aortic balloon is passed through the sheath over the guidewire to a position just below the origin of the left subclavian artery.
- The guidewire is subsequently removed and the catheter lumen is aspirated to remove any residual air or thrombus.
- The intra-aortic balloon is connected to the drive system console and counterpulsation can subsequently begin.
- The augment pressure tracing should be inspected for proper timing in the 1:2 mode (Figure 15.3).
- The intra-aortic balloon catheter and femoral sheath should be secured with sutures.

Timing

Proper timing of balloon inflation and deflation is important because suboptimal timing can lead to hemodynamic instability (Figures 15.4 and 15.5). See Table 15.5 for more information on the impact of timing errors. Many of the currently available catheters are available

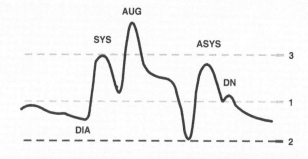

Abbreviation	Definition
DIA	Unassisted End Diastolic Pressure
SYS	Unassisted Peak Systolic Pressure
AUG	Diastolic Augmentation/Peak Diastolic Pressure
ADIA	Assisted End Diastolic Pressure
ASYS	Assisted Peak Systolic Pressure (Systole after IAB deflation)
DN	Dicrotic Notch

Figure 15.3 1:2 IABP inflation. Note that in a 1:2 or 1:3 mode, the SBP that immediately precedes augmentation is actually called the unassisted SBP.

DBP, diastolic blood pressure; IABP, intra-aortic balloon pump; SBP, systolic blood pressure.

Source: Image courtesy of Teleflex Incorporated. © 2013 Teleflex Incorporated. All rights reserved. Retrieved from https://flexlearning.jimdo.com/arrow-support-materials/

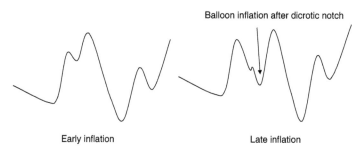

Figure 15.4 Inappropriate timing: Early inflation and late inflation. Late inflation results in suboptimal augmentation.

with fiberoptic manometers that enhance timing. Timing is done with the assist ratio at 1:2 so that you can visualize an augmented or assisted beat and a nonaugmented, or nonassisted, beat. The pump can be programmed to inflate and deflate with each cardiac cycle

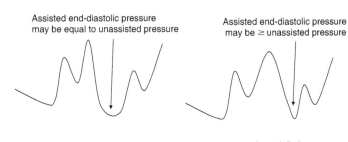

Early deflation

Late deflation

Figure 15.5 Inappropriate timing: Early deflation and late deflation. Early deflation results in suboptimal diastolic augmentation, suboptimal afterload reduction, and a potential for retrograde coronary and carotid flow. Late deflation leads to increased afterload.

Table 15.5

Intra-Aortic Balloon Timing Errors

Early balloon inflation
- Potentially dangerous timing error
- Increases afterload
- Increases myocardial oxygen consumption
- Reduces stroke volume

Early balloon deflation
- Does not decrease afterload
- Reduces time for diastolic filling of coronary arteries

Late balloon inflation
- Reduces time for diastolic filling of coronary arteries

Late balloon deflation
- Very dangerous timing error

Source: Adapted from Jacobson, C., Marzlin, K., & Webner, C. (2014). *Cardiovascular nursing practice: A comprehensive resource manual ad study guide for clinical nurses.* Burien, WA: Cardiovascular Nursing Education Associates.

(1:1 support). Additional assist ratios vary depending on the manufacturer: 1:2, 1:4, 1:8.

- Inflation: The balloon should inflate with the onset of diastole (closure of the aortic valve), which is indicated by the dicrotic notch on the arterial line tracing. This rapid inflation increases the diastolic pressure and displaces blood forward into the aortic root. Coronary arteries fill during diastole, so this additional blood flow increases coronary flow.
- Deflation: The balloon should deflate just before the opening of the aortic valve or the onset of the R wave. This rapid deflation displaces blood, leading to decreased afterload. Additional benefits include decreased myocardial workload and decreased preload.

Essential Facts

- If the patient is having arrhythmias, timing can be challenging. If the patient is markedly tachycardic, you may need to decrease the assist ratio to 1:2.
- Balloon perforation causing helium leak is rare. Blood in the helium gas line indicates balloon rupture. The catheter will need to be removed.
- Pumping failure is also uncommon. If the balloon will not inflate and deflate, check the level of the helium and check all connections. Manual inflation of the balloon will be required to prevent thrombus formation around the catheter.

Potential complications include:

- Vascular injury, bleeding, hematoma
- Limb ischemia
- Aortic dissection, arterial perforation during placement
- Embolic events: gas, plaque, or thrombus
- Thrombocytopenia
- Infection

Ventricular Support Devices

Impella Heart Pump

The Impella heart pump is a short-term percutaneous LV assist device (LVAD). The dual-lumen catheter contains a microaxial continuous flow pump that pulls blood from the LV, displacing it into the ascending aorta. This results in the rapid unloading of the LV and increases forward flow. Table 15.6 compares and contrasts the available features of the available Impella devices.

Indications
- High-risk percutaneous coronary intervention (PCI)
- Cardiogenic shock
- Postcardiotomy pump failure

Contraindications
- Mechanical aortic valve
- Severe AS
- LV thrombus

Complications
- Vascular injury, bleeding, hematoma
- Limb ischemia

Table 15.6

Impella Catheters	
Impella 2.5	Catheter diameter 9 Fr, 12 Fr at the pump motor Flow rate up to 2.5 L/minute Placed percutaneously via the femoral artery and advanced over a guidewire into the ascending aorta, across the aortic valve and into the LV
Impella CP	Catheter diameter 9 Fr, 14 Fr at pump motor Flow rate up to 4.3 L/minute Placed the same as the Impella 2.5
Impella 5.0	Catheter diameter 9 Fr, 21 Fr at pump motor Flow rate up to 5.0 L/minute Placed in the axillary artery or cutdown of the femoral artery and advanced over a guidewire into the ascending aorta, across the aortic valve and into the LV
Impella LD	Catheter diameter 9 Fr, 21 Fr at the pump motor Flow rate up to 5.0 L/minute Placed into the LV during open chest procedure

Fr, French; LV, left ventricle.

- Embolization
- Hemolysis
- Infection

Impella Right Heart Catheter

The Impella RP is designed to provide short-term right heart support by pumping blood from the inferior vena cava to the pulmonary artery to unload the right heart. The 11 Fr catheter (22 Fr at the pump motor) is advanced through a 23 Fr venous sheath with the distal tip in the pulmonary artery. Flow rate is 4.0 L/min.

Indications
- Cardiac surgery
- Cardiac transplant
- Acute myocardial infarction
- Post LVAD placement

Contraindications
- Tricuspid or pulmonary valve stenosis or regurgitation
- Thrombus in the right atrium or vena cava
- Presence of a vena cava filter or vena caval interruption device

Potential Complications

- Arrhythmia
- Bleeding
- Hemolysis
- Infection

TandemHeart

The TandemHeart system is a short-term percutaneous continuous flow LVAD, indicated for the treatment of cardiogenic shock. It can provide up to 4–5 L/min of forward flow. A transseptal approach is required for the placement of this device. Two cannulas are placed: one in the left atrium (LA) via transseptal puncture from the femoral vein and one in the femoral artery. Echocardiographic guidance is used for the placement of the LA cannula. Oxygenated blood is withdrawn from the LA and returned to the femoral artery.

Contraindications

- Coagulopathy
- Severe peripheral arterial disease

Potential Complications

- Vascular injury, bleeding, hematoma
- Limb ischemia
- Cardiac tamponade

Extracorporeal Membrane Oxygenation

There are two types of extracorporeal membrane oxygenation (ECMO): venovenous (VV) and venoarterial (VA). VV-ECMO is primarily used for patients with respiratory failure. VA-ECMO also provides hemodynamic support, so it can be useful for patients with advanced cardiac disease.

In VA-ECMO, the venous cannula is placed in the inferior vena cava or the right atrium. The preferred site for the arterial cannula is the femoral artery. If this is not possible, the right common carotid artery or the axillary artery may be used. Anticoagulation is needed during VA-ECMO therapy. In general, ECMO is a modality provided at larger tertiary hospitals that have specialized teams in place to provide this service. Care of the patient receiving ECMO is complex and beyond the scope of this book.

Indications

- Cardiogenic shock
- Failure to wean from cardiopulmonary bypass following cardiac surgery
- Massive pulmonary embolism
- Cardiac arrest
- Bridge to ventricular assist device
- Bridge to heart transplant

Contraindications

- Known severe brain injury
- Prolonged CPR without adequate tissue perfusion
- Unwitnessed cardiac arrest
- Widespread malignancy
- Severe organ dysfunction

Complications

- Bleeding: Occurs in up to 50% of patients; related to anticoagulation and platelet dysfunction
- Thromboembolism: Related to thrombus formation
- Infection
- Limb ischemia, compartment syndrome
- Cardiac thrombosis
- Neurological injury
- Pulmonary hemorrhage
- Heparin-induced thrombocytopenia (HIT): Can occur due to heparin exposure; confirmed HIT requires change to nonheparin anticoagulation

SUMMARY

Becoming skilled in managing the unstable, decompensating patient comes with experience and exposure. Be familiar with the various medications used to impact heart rate and blood pressure. Practice with the temporary pacemaker generator to gain confidence with its use. Know how to set up and assist with the placement of support devices that are available to you in your setting. Work with your industry partners to get continuing education and updates.

Bibliography

Abbott, J. D. (2017). *Drug-eluting intracoronary stents: General principles.* Retrieved from www.uptodate.com

American Society of Anesthesiologists. (2014). ASA physical status classification system. Retrieved from https://www.asahq.org/resources/clinical-information/asa-physical-status-classification-system

Andreou, C., Maniotis, C., & Koutouzis, M. (2017). The rise and fall of anticoagulation with bivalirudin during percutaneous coronary intervention: A review article. *Cardiology and Therapy, 6,* 1–12. doi:10.1007.s40119-017.0082-x

Apfelbaum, J. L., Gross, J. B., Connis, R. T., Arnold, D. E., Coté, C. J., Dutton, R., . . . Tung, A. (2018). Practice guidelines for moderate procedural sedation and analgesia 2018: A report by the American Society of Anesthesiologists Task Force on Moderate Procedural Sedation and Analgesia, the American Association of Oral and Maxillofacial Surgeons, American College of Radiology, American Dental Association, American Society of Dentist Anesthesiologists, and Society of Interventional Radiology. *Anesthesiology, 128,* 437–479. doi:10.1097/ALN.0000000000002043

Badawy, M. K., Deb, P., Chan, R., & Farouque, O. (2016). A review of radiation protection solutions for the staff in the cardiac catheterisation laboratory. *Heart, Lung, and Circulation, 25,* 961–967. doi:10.1016/j.hlc2016.02.021

Beavers, C. J., & Bagai, J. (2017). *Moderate sedation practices for adult patients in the cardiac catheterization laboratory.* Retrieved from www.scai.org

Bhatt, D. (Ed.). (2016). *Cardiovascular intervention: A companion to Braunwald's heart disease.* Philadelphia, PA: Elsevier.

Burlingame, B., Davidson, J., Denholm, B., Fearon, M. C., Giarrizzo-Wilson, S., Link, T., . . . Wood, A. (2018). *Guidelines for perioperative practice.* R. Conner (Ed.).

Callan, P., & Clark, A. L. (2016). Right heart catheterization: Indications and interpretation. *Heart, 102,* 147–157. doi:10.1136/heartjnl-2015-307786

Carrossa, J. P., & Levin, T. (2017). *Periprocedural complications of percutaneous coronary intervention.* Retrieved from www.uptodate.com

Chau, C. H., & Williams, D. O. (2016). Prevention of contrast induced renal failure for the interventional cardiologist. *Circulation: Cardiovascular Interventions, 9,* e004122. doi:10.1161/CIRCINTERVENTIONS.116.004122

Criscitelli, T. (2018). *Fast facts for the operating room nurse.* New York, NY: Springer Publishing Company, LLC.

Fairman, R. (2018). *Carotid stenting and its complications.* Retrieved from www.uptodate.com

Fazel, R., Gerber, T. C., Balter, S., Brenner, D. J., Carr, J. J., Cerqueira, M. D., . . . Shaw, L. J. (2014). Approaches to enhancing radiation safety in cardiovascular imaging. *Circulation, 130,* 1730–1748. doi:10.1161/CIR.0000000000000048

Gallego, Y., & Rutledge, D. N. (2016). Preventing contrast-induced acute kidney injury. *American Journal of Nursing, 116*(12), 38–44. doi:10.1097/01.NAJ.0000508664.33963.20

Gerhard-Herman, M. D., Gornik, H. L., Barrett, C., Barshes, N. R., Corriere, M. A., Drachman, D. E., . . . Walsh, M. E. (2016). AHA/ACC guideline on the management of patients with lower extremity peripheral artery disease: Executive summary: A report of the American College of Cardiology/American Heart Association Task Force on Clinical Practice Guidelines. *Circulation.* doi:10.1161/CIR.0000000000000470

Hanna, E. B., & Glancy, D. L. (2013). *Practical cardiovascular hemodynamics with self-assessment problems.* New York, NY: Demos Medical Publishing, LLC.

Heidbuchel, H., Wittkamp, F. H. M., Vano, E., Ernst, S., Schilling, R., Picano, E., & Mont, L. (2014). Practical ways to reduce radiation dose for patients and staff during device implantations and electrophysiological procedures. *Europace, 16,* 946–964. doi:10.1093/europace/eut409

Jacobson, C., Marzlin, K., & Webner, C. (2014). *Cardiovascular nursing practice: A comprehensive resource manual ad study guide for clinical nurses.* Burien, WA: Cardiovascular Nursing Education Associates.

The Joint Commission (TJC). (2017). *Sentinel event alert 47: Radiation risks of diagnostic imaging.* Retrieved from https://www.jointcommission.org/sea_issue_47/

Kern, M. J. (2017a). *Cardiac catheterization techniques: Normal hemodynamics.* Retrieved from www.uptodate.com

Kern, M. J. (2017b). *Clinical use of coronary artery pressure flow measurements.* Retrieved from www.uptodate.com

Kern, M. J. (2017c). *Hemodynamics of valvular disorders as measured by cardiac catheterization.* Retrieved from www.uptodate.com

Kern, M. J. (2018). Novel radiation protection devices: An update on radiation safety in the cath lab. *Cath Lab Digest, 26*(1).

Kern, M. J., Lim, M. J., & Sorajia, P. (2018). *The interventional cardiac catheterization handbook* (4th ed.). Philadelphia, PA: Elsevier Saunders.

Kern, M. J., Sorajia, P., & Lim, M. (2016). *The cardiac catheterization handbook* (6th ed.). Philadelphia, PA: Elsevier Saunders.

Khalil, M., & Bagai, J. (2018). *Radiation safety: Are you doing enough to protect yourself and your staff.* Retrieved from www.scai.org

Kumar, G., & Rab, S. T. (2016). *Radiation safety for the interventional cardiologist: A practical approach to protecting ourselves from the dangers of ionizing radiation.* Retrieved from http://www.acc.org/latest-in-cardiology/articles/2015/12/31/10/12/radiation-safety-for-the-interventional-cardiologist

Lee, M. S., & Kong, J. (2015). Achieving safe femoral arterial access. *Current Cardiology Reports, 17*, 44. doi:10.1007s11886-015-0596-6

Levin, T., & Cutlip, D. (2017). *General principles of the use of intracoronary stents.* Retrieved from www.uptodate.com

Lim, S. Y. (2016). No-reflow phenomenon by intracoronary thrombus in acute myocardial infarction. *Chonnam Medical Journal, 52*, 38–44. doi:10.4068/cmj.2016.52.1.38

Lough, M. A. (2016). *Hemodynamic monitoring: Evolving technologies and clinical practice.* St. Louis, MO: Elsevier.

Makdisi, G., & Wang, I. (2015). Extra corporeal membrane oxygenation: Review of a lifesaving technology. *Journal of Thoracic Disease, 7*(7), E166–E176. doi:10.3978/j.issn.2072-1439.2015.07.17

Means, G., End, C., & Kaul, P. (2017). Management of percutaneous coronary intervention complications. *Current Treatment Options in Cardiovascular Medicine, 19*, 25. doi:10.1007/s11936-017-0526-6

Meisinger, Q. C., Stahl, C. M., Andre, M. P., & Newton, I. G. (2016). Radiation protection for the fluoroscopy operator and staff. *American Journal of Radiology*, 745–754. doi:10.2214/AJR.16.16556

Moscucci, M. (2013). *Grossman and Baim's cardiac catheterization, angiography, and intervention* (8th ed.). Philadelphia, PA: Lippincott, Williams, and Wilkins.

Naidu, S. S., Aronow, H. D., Box, L. C., Duffy, P. L., Kolansky, D. M., Kupfer, J. M., . . . Blankenship, J. C. (2016). SCAI expert consensus statement: Best practices in the cardiac catheterization laboratory. *Catheterization and Cardiovascular Interventions.* doi:10.1002/ccd.26551

O'Bleness, M. (2017). Contrast-induced nephropathy: What do we know: A literature analysis. *Cath Lab Digest, 25*(6).

Ozkok, S., & Ozkok, A. (2017). Contrast induced acute kidney injury: A review of practical points. *World Journal of Nephrology, 6*(3), 86–99. doi:10.5527/wjn.v6.i3.86

Partida, R. A., & Yeh, R. W. (2017). Contemporary drug-eluting stent platforms: Design, safety, and clinical efficacy. *Cardiology Clinics, 35*, 281–296. doi:10.1016/j.ccl.2016.12.010

Rajebi, H., & Rajebi, M. R. (2015). Optimizing common femoral access. *Techniques in Vascular and Interventional Radiology, 18*, 76–81. doi:10.1053/j.tvir.2015.04.004

Reskalla, S. H., Stankowski, R. V., Hanna, J., & Kloner, R. A. (2017). Management of no-reflow phenomenon in the catheterization laboratory. *Journal of the American College of Cardiology: Cardiovascular Interventions, 10*(3), 215–223. doi:10.1016/j.jcin.2016.11.059

Bibliography

Sheth, R. A., Walker, G., Saad, W. E., Dariushnia, S. R., Ganguli, S., Hogan, M. J., . . . Nikolic, B. (2014). Quality improvement guidelines for vascular access and closure device use. *Journal of Vascular and Interventional Radiology, 25*, 73–84. doi:10.1016/j.jvir.2013.08.011

Sorajia, P., Borlaug, B. A., Dimas, V., Fang, J. C., Forfia, P. R., Givertz, M. M., . . . Naidu, S. S. (2017). Executive summary of the SCAI/HFSA clinical expert consensus document on the use of invasive hemodynamics for the diagnosis and management of cardiovascular disease. *Catheterization and Cardiovascular Interventions, 89*, 1294–1299. doi:10.1002/ccd.27036

Teleflex Timing Guidelines. Retrieved from http://www.teleflexlearn.com/

Thind, G. S., Parida, R., & Gupta, N. (2015). Pharmacotherapy in the cardiac catheterization laboratory. *Cardiovascular Pharmacology, 4*, 146. doi:10.2147/TCRM.S71927

Thomas, M. P., & Bates, E. R. (2017). *Update on primary PCI for patients with STEMI.* Trends in Cardiovascular Medicine. 2017, 27(2):95-102. doi: 10.1016/j.tcm.2016.06.010

Topol, E. J., & Teirstein, P. S. (Ed.). (2016). *Textbook of interventional cardiology.* Philadelphia, PA: Elsevier.

Weisbord, S. D., Gallagher, M., Jneid, H., Garcia, S., Cass, A., Thwin, S.S., . . . Palevsky, P. M. (2018). Outcomes after angiography with sodium bicarbonate and acetylcysteine. *The New England Journal of Medicine, 378*(7), 603–614. doi:10.1056/NEJMoa1710933

Index